Antique
Medical Instruments

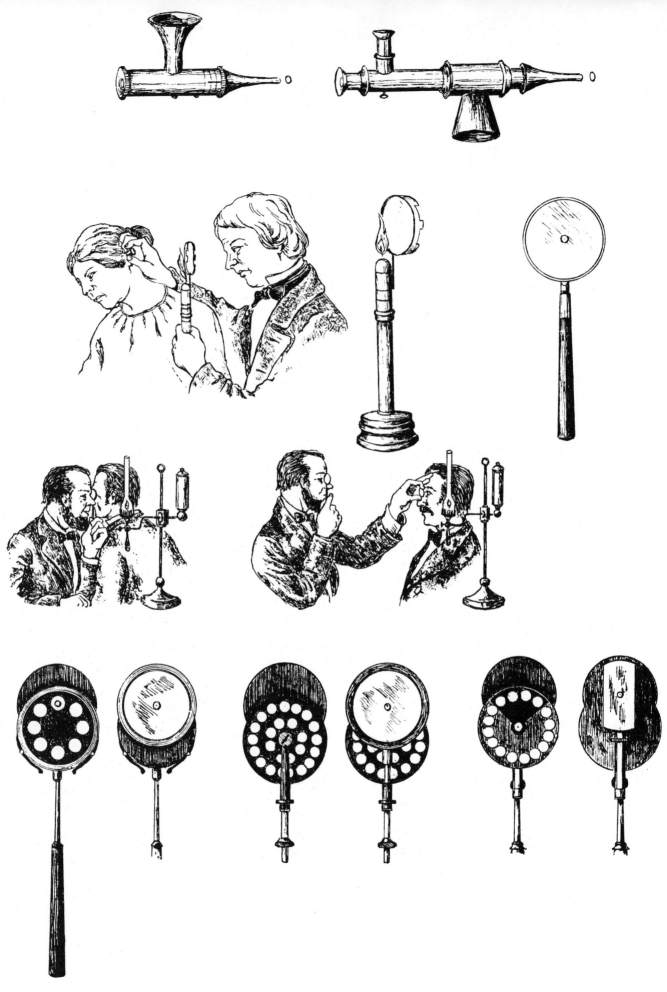

Antique
Medical Instruments

Price Guide Included

C. Keith Wilbur, M.D.

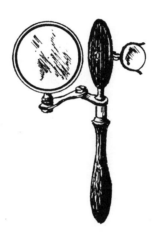

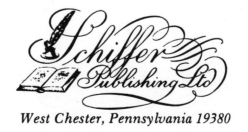

West Chester, Pennsylvania 19380

Printed in the United States of America.
ISBN: 0-88740-094-9
Published by Schiffer Publishing Ltd.
1469 Morstein Road, West Chester, Pennsylvania 19380

This book may be purchased from the publisher.
Please include $2.00 postage.
Try your bookstore first.

Contents

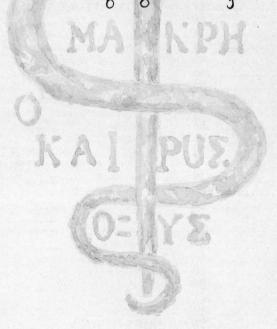

FOREWORD

Some twenty years ago, a patient gifted me with a handsome mahogany box, banded in brass and inscribed U.S.A. The contents were obviously related to my profession — several roundish saws with detached handles, several finely honed scalpels, and some intriguing companion instruments that were head-scratchers. My generous donor wondered how the instruments were used and for what purpose — and when — and I was embarrassed to confess that I had no answers

A modest amount of research proved it to be a Civil War trephining set, pristine and sharp enough to bore into the skull of any unfortunate Union defender. My patient traced the original owner to a New Hampshire army physician who had practiced medicine the best he could with what he had.

Medical instruments represent the very heart of every new diagnostic and therapeutic advance. These innovative and frequently ingenious devices are vital to the ongoing effort to identify disease — and hopefully to bring about a cure.

The following pages focus on the diagnostic tools of the trade that were most frequently used by primary care physicians. Therapeutic instruments will then complete the overview of this long neglected subject.

MICROSCOPES

The early seventeenth century offered two new and vastly different worlds to challenge man's inquisitive and adventurous spirit. The American colonists had their toe-hold in the New World and were gradually expanding from the coastal implants. While back in the mother countries, exploration of an invisible world - quite unknown to the unaided eye - was underway. Crude microscopes were zeroing in on everything from plant cells and butterfly wings to blood cells tumbling about in the thin webbing of a frog's foot. It was a fantasy world that gave little hint of the potential ahead for the physician and his infection-ridden patients.

A few dedicated souls fashioned their own lenses and mounted the glass in some sort of convenient holder. If this were made with a tube that could slide inside another or be provided with a screw thread, the distance between the lenses at both ends could be brought into focus. But except for some drawings of these hidden wonders by such enthusiasts as Robert Hooke their efforts were isolated and usually captured the imagination of the few who could afford such extravagances. For the seventeenth and eighteenth century well-to-do, the microscope became a parlor toy for an evening's entertainment.

Meanwhile the serious investigators continued to observe and wonder over their discoveries. One Athanasius Kircher (1601-1680) even insisted that the microorganisms he saw were the cause of infectious disease. It was an attractive idea, but was soon discredited when others used their imperfect instruments to report fanciful "beasties" that just didn't exist.

On the American front, such nonsense had no place in the real world where a living must be carved from the wilderness. Not until the 1830's did technical advances make the microscope really practical. Then - and only then - did the Americans enter the field of microscopy with enthusiasm.

LENS ABERRATIONS ~ frustrating distortions of images and loss of clarity.

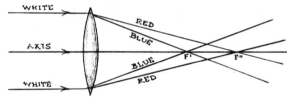

CHROMATIC ABERRATION ~ WAVES OF VARYING LENGTH MAKE UP ORDINARY LIGHT. WHEN PASSED THROUGH A LENS, SHORT WAVES (BLUE) ARE BENT THE MOST AND FOCUS NEAR THE LENS (F'). THE LONG WAVES (RED) FOCUS AT A MORE DISTANT POINT (F"), WHILE INTERMEDIATE RAYS FALL BETWEEN THESE TWO FOCAL POINTS. THIS RESULTS IN AN INDISTINCT HALO OF COLORS AROUND THE IMAGE.

SPHERICAL ABERRATION ~ WHEN A LIGHT RAY PASSES THROUGH A LENS, IT BENDS TOWARD THE THICKEST PART OF THE LENS. MANY RAYS WILL THEREFORE CROSS MANY POINTS ON THE AXIS. THE PERIPHERY OF THE IMAGE WILL BE BLURRED.

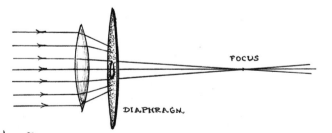

The early microscopes had but one way to block out these renegade rays - with a diaphragm. This disc with a small center hole permitted only those rays near the axial ray to pass. Although the image was sharper, the tiny disc opening effectively cut out most of the necessary light. It was a quandry that the seventeeth and eighteenth century microscope makers pursued - but with little success. Not until the start of the nineteenth century did a combination of lenses with differing dispersive powers - the achromatic lenses - give a single crisp focus without distortion. Until then, the simple microscope generally out-performed its more sophisticated big brother, the compound microscope. Indeed, a majority of the early discoveries were made with -

THE SIMPLE MICROSCOPE.

The simple microscope is nothing more than a bi-convex lens the ordinary magnifying glass fixed on a mount. When the parallel rays from the sun pass through the glass, they bend to meet at the principal focus. If a piece of paper were placed at this point, it would catch afire. Now when an object is placed between the lens and its principal focus, an enlarged upright image is seen. This is a "virtual" image ~ a projection of the retinal image back into the field of vision ~ and doesn't really exist. Unlike the compound microscope, there is no second lens to enlarge this image AND the troublesome aberrations. It is a useful tool where great magnification is not needed.

RETINAL IMAGE

BI-CONVEX LENS

OBJECT WITHIN PRINCIPAL FOCUS

PROJECTED VIRTUAL IMAGE

The lens - the heart of the microscope - increases in power as does its surface curvature. As the curve approaches and becomes a sphere, it reaches its greatest magnification. (Try a clear glass marble to illustrate this point). From here, the only way to increase the power is to make the sphere smaller ~ and the curve thereby greater. Although the old master Leeuwenhoek laboriously ground and polished his lenses, most found the tiny glass globule did a tolerable job in these early microscopes. Robert Hook described the making of these tiny spherical lenses in 1679.

HEAT A SMALL CLEAR GLASS ROD AND DRAW OUT TO A FINE THREAD.

MELT THE END OF THE THREAD TO FORM A SMALL GLASS GLOBULE.

PRICK A SMALL HOLE THROUGH A THIN PLATE OF BRASS OR SILVER. USING THE THREAD AS A HANDLE, FIX THE GLOBULE OVER THE CENTER OF THE HOLE WITH WAX.

PLACE OBJECT ON A JOINTED ARM OR NEEDLE FIXED IN WAX.

SIMPLE MICROSCOPE COMPARISON

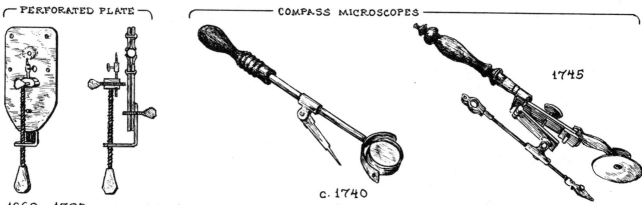

PERFORATED PLATE

COMPASS MICROSCOPES

1745

c. 1740

1668 ~ 1783 LEEUWENHOEK'S FINELY GROUND BI-CONVEX LENSES OPENED OPEN UP THE WORLD OF "ANIMALCULES". SINCE HE MADE A NEW SCOPE FOR EACH PROJECT, OVER 550 WERE COMPLETED. ONLY 9 EXIST TODAY. THE BRASS, SILVER AND EVEN GOLD PLATES ARE TINY ~ LESS THAN 2 INCHES IN HEIGHT AND 1 INCH IN WIDTH!

THE COMPASS MICROSCOPE RESEMBLED A DRAFTSMAN'S COMPASS JOINT. ONE OF THE ARMS WAS A TAPERED PIN, FORCEPS OR LIVE-BOX TO HOLD THE OBJECT FOR VIEWING. ALL WERE HAND-HELD AND THEIR EASE OF USE MADE THEM VERY POPULAR. AVERAGED 6~7 INCHES IN LENGTH. INVENTED BY WILSON 1702.

NOTE ~ MOST OF THE MICROSCOPES ILLUSTRATED ARE FROM THE BILLINGS MICROSCOPE COLLECTION.

SIMPLE MICROSCOPE ~ SCREW ~ BARREL ~ BRASS.

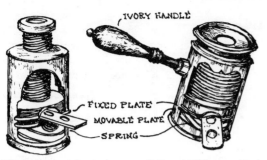

IVORY HANDLE

FIXED PLATE
MOVABLE PLATE
SPRING

1702 WILSON'S FIRST MODEL ~ ENGLISH

1706~1750 WILSON ~ ENGLISH

BASE SPRING PRESSURES LOWER PLATE AGAINST SANDWICHED IVORY SLIDER.

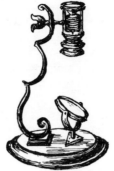

C. 1750 SCROLL PILLAR ~ ENGLISH.

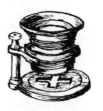

C. 1830 PILLAR WITH PIVOTING LENS TUBE ~ ENGLISH.

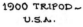

1900 TRIPOD ~ U.S.A.

SIMPLE ~ PILLAR WITH ADJUSTABLE ARM ~ BRASS.

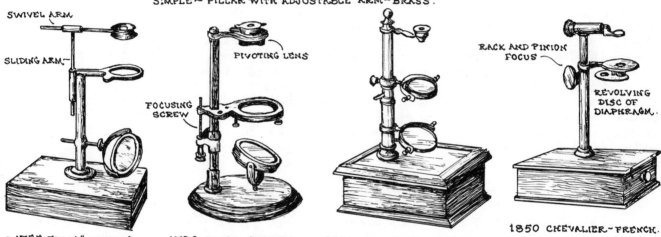

SWIVEL ARM

SLIDING ARM

FOCUSING SCREW

PIVOTING LENS

RACK AND PINION FOCUS

REVOLVING DISC OF DIAPHRAGM.

C. 1755 ELLIS "AQUATIC" ~ ENGLISH.

1798 JONES ~ ENGLISH.

1831 NATURALIST DARWIN'S ~ ENGLISH.

1850 CHEVALIER ~ FRENCH.

"AQUATIC" MOTION MEANT UNLIMITED POSITIONING WITH HORIZONTAL SWIVELING ARM AND VERTICAL PILLAR ADJUSTMENT. MOST WERE PORTABLE AFTER THE PILLAR WAS UNSCREWED AND PLACED IN THE WOODEN BOX BASE. THIS STYLE WAS POPULAR THROUGH THE 1800'S.

SIMPLE DISSECTING MICROSCOPES ~ BRASS.

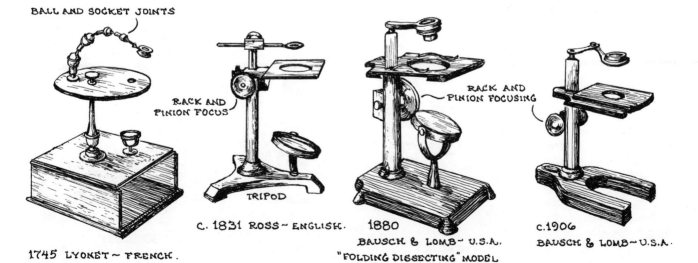

BALL AND SOCKET JOINTS

RACK AND PINION FOCUS

RACK AND PINION FOCUSING

1745 LYONET ~ FRENCH.

C. 1831 ROSS ~ ENGLISH.

1880 BAUSCH & LOMB ~ U.S.A. "FOLDING DISSECTING" MODEL

c.1906 BAUSCH & LOMB ~ U.S.A.

THE COMPOUND MICROSCOPE ~ MONOCULAR

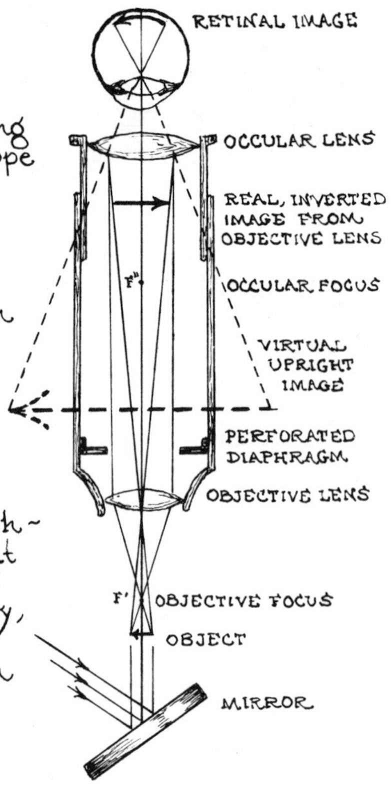

Some unsung Dutch observer in the early seventeenth century found that magnification could be increased by adding a second lens (the objective) to that of the simple microscope (occular or eye lens). The compound (several lens systems) monocular (for use with one eye) microscope had begun its long and invaluable career.

Briefly, the objective lens forms a "real" image ~ one where the light rays from the object actually passes through the lens. To do so, the object studied must be placed at a distance further from the lens than its focal length (to F'). The object image will be inverted when further enlarged by the occular lens ~ if the image falls between the occular lens and its focal point at F". The eye will see this as a greatly enlarged virtual and right-side-up image.

As noted, the early compound microscope was not without problems. The chromatic and spherical aberrations that plagued pioneer investigators were somewhat reduced by an internal diaphragm with a small central opening. Unfortunately, so was the light coming from the object. Reflected light from a tilting mirror was of some help. But the big breakthrough came in the late 1820's when achromatic microscope lenses made the diaphragm obsolete. Ten years later it was back as a part of the new and revolutionary achromatic condenser. It's iris ~ like action could regulate the concentrated light from this substage condenser. Image distortion and poor lighting no longer hindered future discoveries.

(diagram labels, top right)
RETINAL IMAGE
OCCULAR LENS
REAL, INVERTED IMAGE FROM OBJECTIVE LENS
OCCULAR FOCUS
VIRTUAL UPRIGHT IMAGE
PERFORATED DIAPHRAGM
OBJECTIVE LENS
F' OBJECTIVE FOCUS
OBJECT
MIRROR

COMPOUND MICROSCOPE COMPARISON

Imitation has long been the sincerest form of flattery among the microscope makers. Each borrowed freely and without apologies from the latest improvements in the field. Still, two separate inventive thrusts were evident ~ the English and the European Continental styles. By the mid nineteenth century, the Americans elbowed their way into the competition. In keeping with tradition, our country was soon producing high quality instruments with features from both the English and Continental microscopes.

ENGLISH STYLES

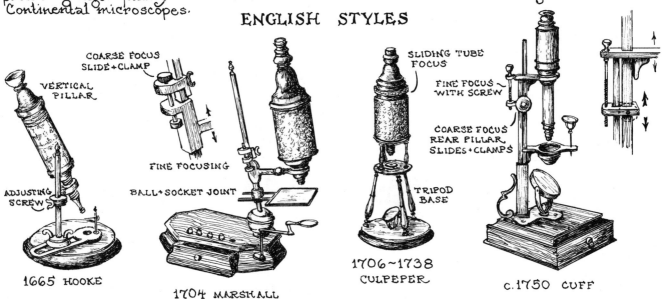

VERTICAL PILLAR
ADJUSTING SCREWS
1665 HOOKE

COARSE FOCUS SLIDE + CLAMP
FINE FOCUSING
BALL + SOCKET JOINT
1704 MARSHALL

SLIDING TUBE FOCUS
1706~1738 CULPEPER
TRIPOD BASE

FINE FOCUS ~ WITH SCREW
COARSE FOCUS REAR PILLAR SLIDES + CLAMPS
c.1750 CUFF

Although the American physician remained unimpressed by the increased interest in microscopy across the seas, there were those institutions that gave these new gadgets a try. Padgitt reports that Yale imported a Culpeper model in 1734, Harvard a screw-barrel-perhaps simple-in 1732 plus a Nairne chest model in 1792, and Brown University several compound microscopes by 1769. Meanwhile, the upright sliding brass pillars with improved focusing and inclination continued to be characteristic of the English eighteenth century effort.

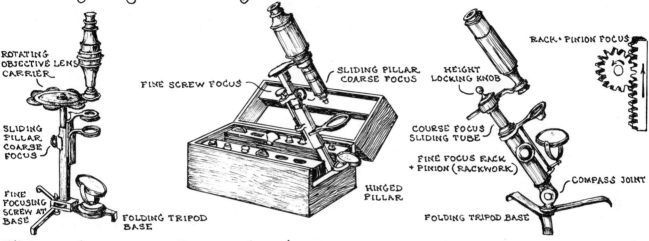

ROTATING OBJECTIVE LENS CARRIER

SLIDING PILLAR COARSE FOCUS

FINE FOCUSING SCREW AT BASE

FOLDING TRIPOD BASE

1746 ADAMS' "NEW UNIVERSAL DOUBLE"

FINE SCREW FOCUS

SLIDING PILLAR COARSE FOCUS

HINGED PILLAR

1760 NAIRNE "CHEST" PORTABLE MICROSCOPE
~ POPULAR WELL INTO NINETEENTH CENTURY ~

RACK + PINION FOCUS

HEIGHT LOCKING KNOB

COURSE FOCUS SLIDING TUBE

FINE FOCUS RACK + PINION (RACKWORK)

COMPASS JOINT

FOLDING TRIPOD BASE

1776 MARTIN'S "NEW UNIVERSAL"

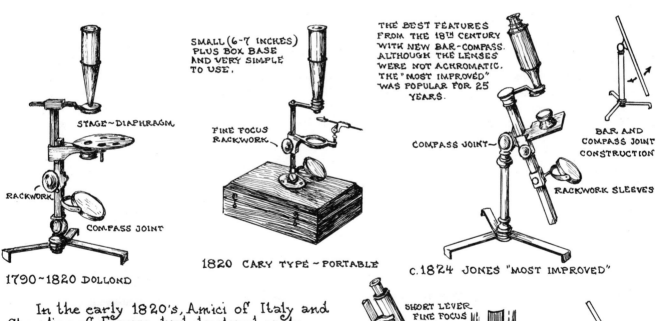

STAGE~DIAPHRAGM

RACKWORK

COMPASS JOINT

1790~1820 DOLLOND

SMALL (6-7 INCHES) PLUS BOX BASE AND VERY SIMPLE TO USE.

FINE FOCUS RACKWORK

1820 CARY TYPE ~ PORTABLE

THE BEST FEATURES FROM THE 18TH CENTURY WITH NEW BAR-COMPASS. ALTHOUGH THE LENSES WERE NOT ACHROMATIC, THE "MOST IMPROVED" WAS POPULAR FOR 25 YEARS.

COMPASS JOINT

BAR AND COMPASS JOINT CONSTRUCTION

RACKWORK SLEEVES

c.1824 JONES "MOST IMPROVED"

In the early 1820's, Amici of Italy and Chevalier of France had developed early achromatic objective lens combinations. By combining a crown glass convex lens with a concave lens of flint glass, aberrations markedly decreased.

In 1830, Lister of England took the achromatic lens out of the trial and error method by calculating the lens corrections for truly achromatic lens- a milestone in microscopy.

SHORT LEVER FINE FOCUS

"LISTER" LIMB

AMONG LISTER'S CONTRIBUTION WAS THE "LISTER" LIMB TO GIVE STURDINESS AND STABILITY TO THE MICROSCOPE STAND.

1839 ROSS

A small point, but the 1839 Ross used glass slides instead of the time-honored ivory specimen sliders on the stage.

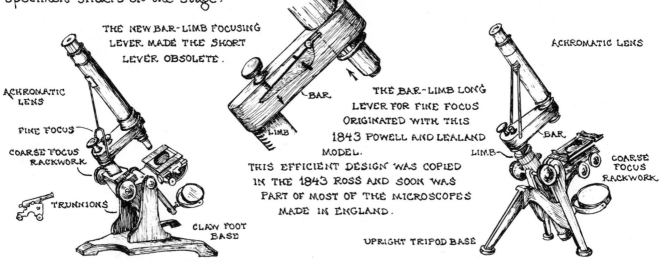

THE NEW BAR-LIMB FOCUSING LEVER MADE THE SHORT LEVER OBSOLETE.

ACHROMATIC LENS

FINE FOCUS

COARSE FOCUS RACKWORK

TRUNNIONS

CLAW FOOT BASE

1843 ROSS

BAR

LIMB

THE BAR-LIMB LONG LEVER FOR FINE FOCUS ORIGINATED WITH THIS 1843 POWELL AND LEALAND MODEL.
THIS EFFICIENT DESIGN WAS COPIED IN THE 1843 ROSS AND SOON WAS PART OF MOST OF THE MICROSCOPES MADE IN ENGLAND.

UPRIGHT TRIPOD BASE

ACHROMATIC LENS

BAR

LIMB

COARSE FOCUS RACKWORK

1843 POWELL AND LEALAND

For the remainder of the century, the "Lister"-limb and the bar-limb were found on the best instruments that the English had to offer. Beginning with Powell's 1841 microscope, most had achromatic substage condensers to concentrate an undistorted light on the objective. Expensive indeed, but of a quality that would make them of use in the medicine of today.

THE CONTINENTAL STYLE

Back in 1738, Englishman Ben Martin hit upon a design that would inspire generations of European instrument makers. This "pocket" microscope was indeed portable, and little more than a cardboard tube and a turned wooden eye cone. Just a handy six inches in length, Martin even suggested that it could be screwed into the hollow handle of a walking stick or whip! Gradually the tube evolved into the drum base and later the familiar horseshoe base. By 1890, most American microscopes had discarded the English features in favor of the Continental — and the style persists today.

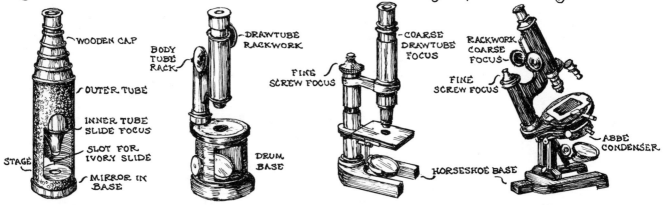

WOODEN CAP

OUTER TUBE

INNER TUBE SLIDE FOCUS

SLOT FOR IVORY SLIDE

STAGE

MIRROR IN BASE

1738 MARTIN, ENGLISH

BODY TUBE RACK

DRAWTUBE RACKWORK

DRUM BASE

1840 OBERHAUSER, FRANCE

COARSE DRAWTUBE FOCUS

FINE SCREW FOCUS

HORSESHOE BASE

c.1885 LEITZ, GERMANY
A SMALL CONTINENTAL STAND

RACKWORK COARSE FOCUS

FINE SCREW FOCUS

ABBÉ CONDENSER

1891 ZEISS, GERMANY
A LARGE CONTINENTAL STAND

For a century and a half, Continental enthusiasts were happy enough to brighten their objects with a concave mirror and a substage wheel of diaphragms. Until 1870, that is. Ernst Abbe, working with Zeiss, proved that his substage condenser was a necessity.

ZEISS ACHROMATIC CONDENSER, CUT AWAY TO SHOW THE COMBINATION OF LENSES.

This new illuminator, inexpensive and free of distortion, became the constant companion of most later microscopes.

MADE IN AMERICA

The microscope and its dim, blurred objects with colored halos had left the Americans uninspired. Then in 1830, fellow countryman Edward Thomas published his thoughts for better microscopy ~ and others sat up and took notice. For one thing, he stated that the image quality was far worse with spherical aberration than chromatic aberration. Also blue light gave better resolution than broad daylight. And he determined that the larger the adjustable opening (aperture) of the objective lens, the clearer the details of an object to be studied. Not exactly a thunderbolt, but it did set the scientific community to considering the optical possibilities.

Ten years later, Charles Spencer began turning out microscopes with superior optical lenses. Since there was a wide choice of mechanically efficient stands in both the English and Continental tradition, his ~ and most of the other early American makers ~ products resembled the external features of that period.

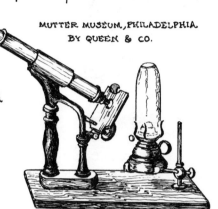

MUTTER MUSEUM, PHILADELPHIA
BY QUEEN & CO.

Meanwhile, Dr. Oliver Wendell Holmes had completed his Paris studies in 1835. He returned to Harvard Medical School with a microscope and promptly started America's first course in microscopy. When he became Professor of Anatomy and Physiology in 1847, he fitted an attic space in the medical building as the "Microscope Room". Still later, he found his lectures could be better illustrated by a special ~ and very inexpensive ~ microscope of his own design. The instrument could be passed from one student to another to actually view the tissue under discussion.

1873 HOLMES CLASS MICROSCOPE

ORIGINS OF AMERICAN DESIGN

CHEVALIER 1827 ⟶ SPENCER 1840~1850

The appearance of the horozontal microscope was brief ~ but spectacular. Meant for better viewing when seated, it first housed an ingenious reflecting mirror to enlarge and reflect an image that was free from distortion.

Amici of Italy had the idea in 1820, and it worked well enough if the mirror were carefully crafted and perfectly alligned in the optical axis of the barrel.

The reflecting microscope faded into history when Amici and Chevalier of France combined efforts to produce ~ at last! ~ a truly achromatic micoscope ~ the 1827 "Universal". Although the achromatic lens combination was discovered by trial-and-error (Lister would shortly spell out an optical formula for achromatic lenses) it was quite efficient. The design was still in the horozontal, but by pivoting the arm on the compass joint and removing the nosepiece, the microscope could be converted to the vertical. Quite "universal".

HOROZONTAL POSITION

1840-50 SPENCER

VERTICAL

1840-50 SPENCER

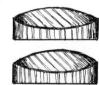

1825 CHEVALIER'S ACHROMATIC OBJECTIVES COMBINATION.

America's first microscope by Charles Spencer in the 1840s was based on Chevalier's horozontal-to-vertical style. Only the focusing arrangement differed ~ and the addition of Spencer's excellent achromatic lens system.

Before 1885, the English influence on our compound microscope stands was evident with the tripod or claw foot bases, "Lister"-limb or bar-limb and short or long fine focusing mechanisms. Competition was keen, and England and America outdid themselves with large, brassy, complex instruments that were encrusted with knobs, dials and accessories. Between 1880~1890, America changed directions in favor of a simple microscope with an affordable price tag. The Continental design became our standard as the following brief comparison indicates.

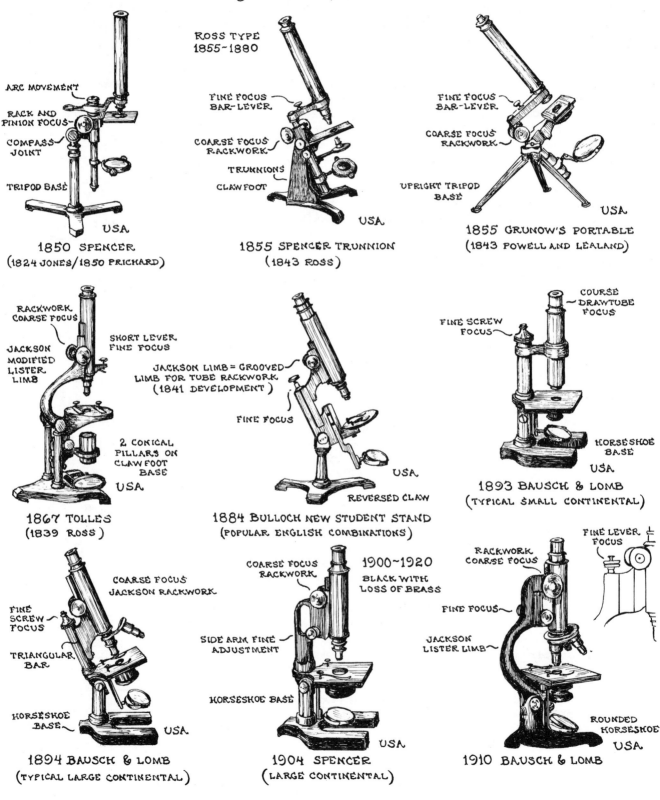

ROSS TYPE 1855~1880

ARC MOVEMENT
RACK AND PINION FOCUS
COMPASS JOINT
TRIPOD BASE
USA
1850 SPENCER
(1824 JONES/1850 PRICHARD)

FINE FOCUS BAR-LEVER
COARSE FOCUS RACKWORK
TRUNNIONS
CLAW FOOT
USA
1855 SPENCER TRUNNION
(1843 ROSS)

FINE FOCUS BAR-LEVER
COARSE FOCUS RACKWORK
UPRIGHT TRIPOD BASE
USA
1855 GRUNOW'S PORTABLE
(1843 POWELL AND LEALAND)

RACKWORK COARSE FOCUS
JACKSON MODIFIED LISTER LIMB
SHORT LEVER FINE FOCUS
2 CONICAL PILLARS ON CLAW FOOT BASE
USA
1867 TOLLES
(1839 ROSS)

JACKSON LIMB = GROOVED LIMB FOR TUBE RACKWORK (1841 DEVELOPMENT)
FINE FOCUS
USA
REVERSED CLAW
1884 BULLOCH NEW STUDENT STAND
(POPULAR ENGLISH COMBINATIONS)

FINE SCREW FOCUS
COURSE DRAWTUBE FOCUS
HORSESHOE BASE
USA
1893 BAUSCH & LOMB
(TYPICAL SMALL CONTINENTAL)

COARSE FOCUS JACKSON RACKWORK
FINE SCREW FOCUS
TRIANGULAR BAR
HORSESHOE BASE
USA
1894 BAUSCH & LOMB
(TYPICAL LARGE CONTINENTAL)

COARSE FOCUS RACKWORK
1900~1920
BLACK WITH LOSS OF BRASS
SIDE ARM FINE ADJUSTMENT
HORSESHOE BASE
USA
1904 SPENCER
(LARGE CONTINENTAL)

RACKWORK COARSE FOCUS
FINE LEVER FOCUS
FINE FOCUS
JACKSON LISTER LIMB
ROUNDED HORSESHOE
USA
1910 BAUSCH & LOMB

AMERICAN ORIGINALS ~
Not all the nineteenth century microscopes from this country were copies or improvements on foreign designs. J.L. Riddell, Professor at the University of Louisiana, discovered a unique optical principle in 1851. If two prisms are placed above the objective lens the light is split to send an image to the two eyepiece tubes. The binocular microscope, much favored today over the monocular or single eye-tube, was an outstanding contribution to the field. Another professor, J. Laurence

USA

1853 RIDDELL'S BINOCULAR
MICROSCOPE BY GRUNOW BROTHERS

USA

1855 SMITH'S INVERTED
BY GRUNOW BROTHERS

Smith of Ohio's Kenyon College, invented the "Chemical or Inverted" microscope. Its unconventional shape allowed the observation of chemical tests without the fumes injuring or clouding the objective lenses.

AMERICAN MICROSCOPE MAKERS

ACME OPTICAL WORKS 1880-1881, Lancaster, Pa. Acquired by QUEEN & COMPANY in 1881, manufacturing the ACME line through 1891 in Philadelphia.

ALLEN, J.B. c 1849, Springfield, Mass.

BAUSCH & LOMB OPTICAL COMPANY 1876 to the present. Rochester, N.Y.

BULLOCH 1864-1866 (optics) N.Y.C.~ BULLOCH 1866-1891, Chicago, Ill.

DALTON 1883-1895, Boston, Mass. TOLLES successor.

FASOLDT 1888-? Albany, N.Y.

GUNDLACH MANHATTAN OPTICAL COMPANY 1879-1884. Became GUNDLACH OPTICAL COMPANY 1884-c.1900.

GRUNOW BROTHERS (or J. & W. GRUNOW or J. & W. GRUNOW & COMPANY) c.1852-1864, New Haven, Conn. and 1864-1874, N.Y.C ~ J. GRUNOW 1874-1892, N.Y.C.

HAWKINS & WALE c.1870-1878, Hoboken, N.J.

KLEINE c.1879-c.1882, N.Y.C.

McALLISTER c.1867-1890's, N.Y.C.

McINTOSH 1872- c.1893, Chicago, Ill.

MILLER BROTHERS 1867 ~ later MILLER AND BROTHER to 1899, N.Y.C.

PIKE'S SON & COMPANY 1878-1883, N.Y.C.

SCHRAUER 1877-1890's, N.Y.C.

SPENCER c.1838-1854, Canastota, N.Y.~ SPENCER AND EATON 1854-c.1865, Canastota, N.Y.~ C.A. SPENCER AND SONS c 1865-1873, Canastota, N.Y. ~ C.A. SPENCER & SONS FOR GENEVA OPTICAL COMPANY 1875-1877, Geneva, N.Y.~ C.A. SPENCER & SONS IN GENEVA 1877-1880, Geneva, N.Y.~ H.R. SPENCER & COMPANY 1880-1888, then moved 1889-1890, Cleveland, Ohio~ SPENCER & SMITH OPTICAL COMPANY 1891-1895, Buffalo, N.Y. ~ SPENCER LENS COMPANY 1895-1935, Buffalo, N.Y. Acquired by AMERICAN OPTICAL COMPANY in 1935 and continues as AMERICAN OPTICAL COMPANY'S SCIENTIFIC INSTRUMENT DIVISION, Buffalo, N.Y.

TOLLES c.1858-1867, Canastota, N.Y ~ Then as BOSTON OPTICAL WORKS 1867-1895, Boston, Mass.

SIDLE, JOHN and PROFESSOR J.E. SMITH 1878, Lancaster, Pa.~ SIDLE AND POALK c.1878-1881 became ACME OPTICAL WORKS 1884-1881.

ZENTMAYER c.1853-1895+, Philadelphia, Pa.

The twentieth century microscope designs remained essentially unchanged except for refinements, interchangable parts and improved accessories.

c.1930 BAUSCH & LOMB BINOCULAR

PHYSICAL DIAGNOSIS

Dr. William Douglass arrived in Boston in 1718 to hang out his shingle. He recalled in his Settlements in North America, "When I first arrived in New England, I asked a noted and facetious practitioner what was their general method of treatment. He told me it was uniformly bleeding, blistering, purging, anodynes, etc. If the illness continued, there was repetendi and finally murderandi."

The practice of medicine in the colonies was clearly patterned after the teaching of the English and continental greats. There was no want of disease theories, with most revolving about an imbalance of bodily fluids or excessive stimulation of the nerves controlling muscles and blood vessels. By quizzing and casually observing the patient, these imbalances or excesses would be evident in such symptoms as fever, rashes, aches and pains, diarrhea and the like. The Boston physician was simply following the time-honored treatment of these symptoms. Such comfortable theories required no time-consuming examinations, only a cookbook approach that would match symptoms with treatment.

Meanwhile, microscopy was giving physicians food for thought. Actual visualization of both healthy and diseased tissues cried out for more attention to the patient himself. The anatomists were also making themselves known with their meticulous dissection of the human body. In 1761 Giovanni Morgagni published The Seats and Causes of Disease Investigated by Anatomy. In this remarkable work, he related pathology found at autopsy to observations made on the living patient. Although the traditional theories would die a slow death, a more scientific view encouraged a hand's-on examination for a surer diagnosis of the patient's disease. Surgeons had necessarily done so for centuries.

PERCUSSION

In 1761, the same year that Morgagni's treatise came into print, there appeared a monograph, "New Invention to Detect the Diseases Hidden Deep Inside the Chest." An elated Austrian physician was sharing his discovery of percussion on the living human chest. It had long been common knowledge that the fluid level of a partially filled wine cask could be determined by tapping. Leopold Auebrugger pondered this, then tried the technique on his own patients. When he struck the healthy chest with the palmar surface of the fingers, it answered with clear, hollow drumlike sounds. But, as with the wine in the cask, pleural fluid or an infected, congested lung yielded only a dull flat "thunk." Further, there was a sense of resistance to the percussing fingers over these diseased areas. He recommended wearing a leather glove or pulling the patient's shirt snuggly to eliminate skin-to-skin noises.

Here was a diagnostic technique that was simplicity itself, yet Auebrugger's "New Invention" met with ho-hums in the theory oriented medical community. Fortunately, percussion was remembered and revived by Napoleon's personal physician, Jean-Nicolas Corvisart. By his example and through his writings, the direct or "immediate" percussion became popular on both sides of the Atlantic. With the American Revolution behind them, our physicians seemed eager for any revolutionary changes in physical diagnosis.

THE PLEXIMETER = "I strike"

Pierre Piorry of Paris was in agreement. He devised a flat disc of polished ivory, about two inches in length and an inch in its greatest width. This first pleximeter was to be held on the chest by means of two upright half inch ears. Its surface was struck with the fingers, and considered "mediate" percussion because of the interposed disc. It was felt to give better resonance over fatty tissue and the intercostal depressions, as well as some patient protection from heavy handed physicians.

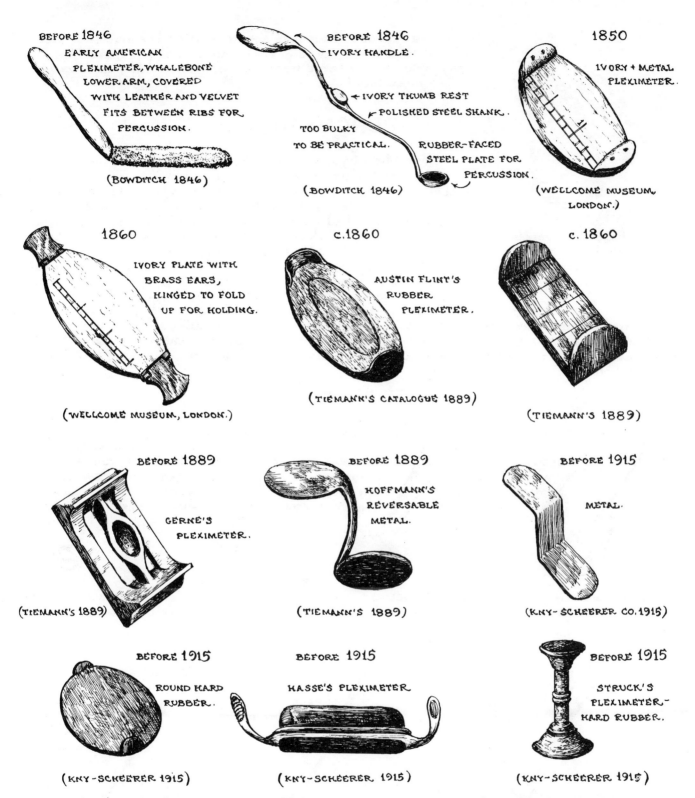

BEFORE 1846
EARLY AMERICAN PLEXIMETER, WHALEBONE LOWER ARM, COVERED WITH LEATHER AND VELVET FITS BETWEEN RIBS FOR PERCUSSION.
(BOWDITCH 1846)

BEFORE 1846
IVORY HANDLE.
← IVORY THUMB REST
← POLISHED STEEL SHANK.
TOO BULKY TO BE PRACTICAL.
RUBBER-FACED STEEL PLATE FOR PERCUSSION.
(BOWDITCH 1846)

1850
IVORY + METAL PLEXIMETER.
(WELLCOME MUSEUM, LONDON.)

1860
IVORY PLATE WITH BRASS EARS, HINGED TO FOLD UP FOR HOLDING.
(WELLCOME MUSEUM, LONDON.)

c.1860
AUSTIN FLINT'S RUBBER PLEXIMETER.
(TIEMANN'S CATALOGUE 1889)

c.1860
(TIEMANN'S 1889)

BEFORE 1889
GERNE'S PLEXIMETER.
(TIEMANN'S 1889)

BEFORE 1889
HOFFMANN'S REVERSABLE METAL.
(TIEMANN'S 1889)

BEFORE 1915
METAL.
(KNY-SCHEERER CO. 1915)

BEFORE 1915
ROUND HARD RUBBER.
(KNY-SCHEERER 1915)

BEFORE 1915
HASSE'S PLEXIMETER
(KNY-SCHEERER 1915)

BEFORE 1915
STRUCK'S PLEXIMETER- HARD RUBBER.
(KNY-SCHEERER 1915)

Austin Flint, America's guiding light on percussion and auscultation, preferred a thin layer of soft India-rubber or wash-leather over the pleximeter's upper surface to avoid extraneous percussion noises. Better yet, he found a square block of India-rubber answers tolerably well." Be that as it may, he noted in 1866 that American physicians preferred their own first or second finger against the chest as a pleximeter. He concluded that such a technique could be used over the ribs and intercostal spaces, was less formidable to the patient (who wasn't used to all that poking and pounding) gave the physician a sense of resistance, cost nothing and was "always at hand."

PERCUSSORS

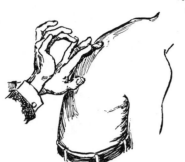

AMERICAN PERCUSSION PREFERANCE ─ ONLY THE THIRD LEFT FINGER CONTACTS THE BODY. THE RIGHT HAND MOVES FROM THE WRIST.

For the physician with bruised fingers, Flint recommended a hammer of India rubber, fixed in a metal ring which in turn was attached to a handle. In his earlier 1856 text, he made note of Bigelow's (Boston) "ball of worsted covered with velvet," Trousseu's (Paris) "thin rod of whalebone with a conical natural rubber", and Marsh's (Dublin) "stethoscope with an India rubber ring surrounding the ear piece". Even Laennac used his cylindrical stethoscope for direct chest percussion ─ a formidable weapon. With this early momentum, the latter half of the nineteenth century exploded with all manner of percussion hammers. But once again Flint reminded his readers that "most practitioners, however, are satisfied with one or more fingers of the right hand, bent in a half circle; and percussion thus made answers all practical purposes." And so it does today.

EARLY PERCUSSORS

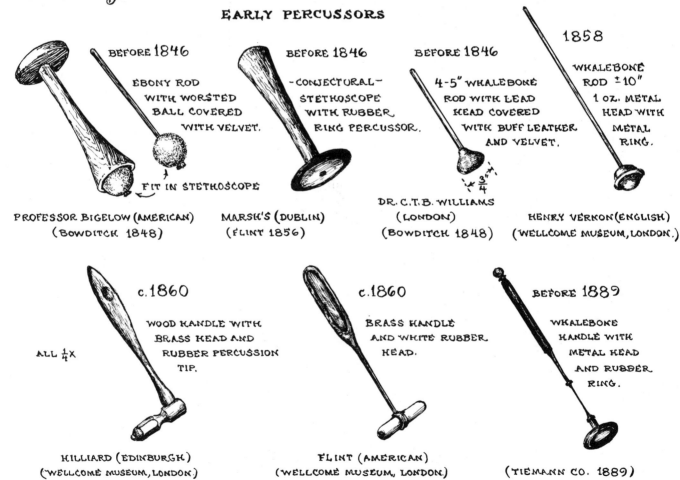

BEFORE 1846

EBONY ROD WITH WORSTED BALL COVERED WITH VELVET.

← FIT IN STETHOSCOPE

PROFESSOR BIGELOW (AMERICAN) (BOWDITCH 1848)

BEFORE 1846

─CONJECTURAL─ STETHOSCOPE WITH RUBBER RING PERCUSSOR.

MARSH'S (DUBLIN) (FLINT 1856)

BEFORE 1846

4-5" WHALEBONE ROD WITH LEAD HEAD COVERED WITH BUFF LEATHER AND VELVET.

$\frac{3}{4}$

DR. C.T.B. WILLIAMS (LONDON) (BOWDITCH 1848)

1858

WHALEBONE ROD ±10" 1 OZ. METAL HEAD WITH METAL RING.

HENRY VERNON (ENGLISH) (WELLCOME MUSEUM, LONDON.)

ALL $\frac{1}{4}$X

c.1860

WOOD HANDLE WITH BRASS HEAD AND RUBBER PERCUSSION TIP.

HILLIARD (EDINBURGH) (WELLCOME MUSEUM, LONDON.)

c.1860

BRASS HANDLE AND WHITE RUBBER HEAD.

FLINT (AMERICAN) (WELLCOME MUSEUM, LONDON.)

BEFORE 1889

WHALEBONE HANDLE WITH METAL HEAD AND RUBBER RING.

(TIEMANN CO. 1889)

REFLEX HAMMERS

In America, the chest percussor was largely ignored~ until 1875, that is. Germany's Wilhelm Erb had been pondering the knee jerk and its possibilities for other than an occasional parlor game. After trial and many errors, he found that almost any muscle in the body would contract involuntarily and instantly if its tendon were stretched by a hammer. Not only that ~ if the patient suffered from a spinal injury or disease, the knee jerk was exceptionally brisk. By 1875, Erb postulated his tendon reflex theory that a nerve arc must carry an impulse from the stimulated tendon to the spinal cord and back to the tendon's muscle to produce an almost instantaneous contraction.

SIMPLE REFLEX ARC ~
THE KNEE JERK IS DIMINISHED OR ABSENT WITH DISEASE AT THIS LEVEL ~ OR INCREASED WITH DISEASE ABOVE THE REFLE LEVEL IN THE SPINE OR BRAIN.

Laboratory confirmation was not long in coming. In Russia, Chiriev experimented with rabbits to prove that when the spinal cord was severed at the origin of the femoral nerve, the knee jerk was absent. The reflex was effectively interrupted. But if the cord were severed above this level and the reflex arc left intact, the knee jerk was increased. Therefore, as Erb suspected, a tendon reflex could pinpoint the level of disease or injury in the spinal cord. Microscopists added to the evidence by identifying the sensory and motor nerves that made up the reflex cycle. Although other nerve pathways also sent the impulse to the brain, the reflex needed no considered response.

Neurology had become of age. Unlike the unproven theories of previous centuries, the simple reflex arc was a solid fact ~ and an aid to physical diagnosis. The old chest percussion hammers were dusted off and put to work stretching tendons. In addition, they saw service when localizing tenderness over the vertebrae, spinous processes, lumbosacral and sacroiliac joints.

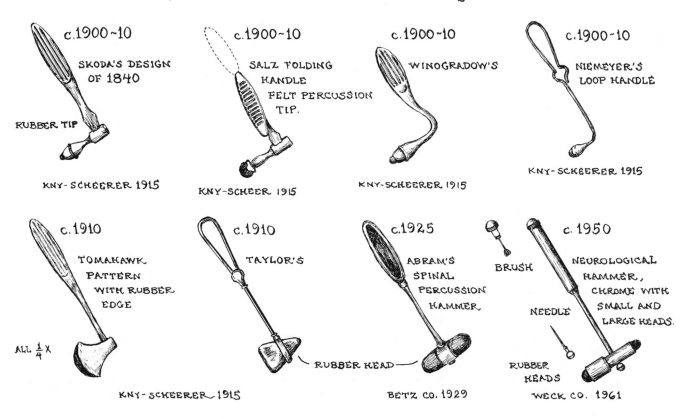

c.1900~10
SKODA'S DESIGN OF 1840
RUBBER TIP
KNY-SCHEERER 1915

c.1900~10
SALZ FOLDING HANDLE
FELT PERCUSSION TIP.
KNY-SCHEER 1915

c.1900~10
WINOGRADOW'S
KNY-SCHEERER 1915

c.1900-10
NIEMEYER'S LOOP HANDLE
KNY-SCHEERER 1915

c.1910
TOMAHAWK PATTERN WITH RUBBER EDGE
ALL ¼ X
KNY-SCHEERER 1915

c.1910
TAYLOR'S
RUBBER HEAD
KNY-SCHEERER 1915

c.1925
ABRAM'S SPINAL PERCUSSION HAMMER
BETZ CO. 1929

c.1950
BRUSH
NEEDLE
NEUROLOGICAL HAMMER, CHROME WITH SMALL AND LARGE HEADS.
RUBBER HEADS
WECK CO. 1961

STETHOSCOPE = Greek "chest" and "I view".

The anatomists had honed their dissecting knives to a fine edge to reveal the disease that had claimed the patient. The microscopist focused in on sections of the abnormal tissue until no detail of pathology escaped their probing lenses. But it was all after the fact, and it was high time that the living patient's problems be discovered objectively ~ well before a visit to the post-mortem slab. The physical examination took on new importance with percussion. But it was a French physician who set the medical profession on its ear with the discovery of the century.

René Laennec had been a valued student of Corvisart and had learned percussion from a master. Inspired, he concentrated on chest diseases and correlated his percussion and ear-to-chest findings with the subsequent autopsy. Laennec was becoming known as an astute diagnostician.

In 1816, the thirtyfive year old physician was examining a young woman with a baffling heart problem. She was stout and well endowed - qualities that frustrated his percussion techniques. Painfully shy, he could not bring himself to press his ear to her chest - the only method of auscultation known. In despiration, he recalled the childhood trick of scratching the end of a log with a pin. The sound would be transmitted loud and clear to a listener at the other end.

Laennec made a sort of laminated "log" on the spot by rolling a quire (one quire = 24 sheets) of writing paper into a compact cylinder. The experiment was an unqualified success. In his words he "··· applied one end of it to the region of the heart and the other to my ear, and was not a little surprised and pleased to find that I could thereby perceive the action of the heart in a manner much more clear and distinct than I had ever been able to do by the immediate application of the ear." In addition, the young lady's modesty remained intact.

This success was followed by a solid wooden cylinder. Further experiments produced a tube with a drilled center, for it was felt that the vibrating air augmented that of the wood.

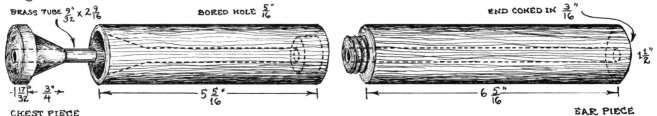

BRASS TUBE $\frac{9}{32}$" x 2$\frac{9}{16}$ BORED HOLE $\frac{5}{16}$"   END CORED IN $\frac{3}{16}$"

$\frac{17}{32}$" $\frac{3}{4}$"   5$\frac{5}{16}$"   6$\frac{5}{16}$"   1$\frac{1}{2}$"

CHEST PIECE   EAR PIECE
MONAURAL STETHOSCOPE MADE BY LAENNAC c. 1819.   (MUTTER MUSEUM, PHILADELPHIA.)
THE PLUG AT THE CHEST END WAS FOR LISTENING TO THE HEART. WHEN REMOVED, THE LARGER OPENING
AUSCULTATED THE LUNG. FOR CLOSER LISTENING, THE HALVES OF THE STETHOSCOPE COULD BE UNSCREWED.

In 1819 Laennec published his," On Mediate Auscultation ~ a classification of all cardiac and respiratory sounds," With it came an unusual bonus ~ a hand-turned wooden cylindrical stethoscope by the author himself! His stethoscopic diagnosis in each recorded case was verified at autopsy, yet there was no sudden stampede for his remarkable listening instrument. Many of the old guard, unable to sort out the rumbles, wheezes and murmurs enhanced by the stethoscope, defended the ear-on-chest or "immediate" auscultation. But in spite of such obstructionists, the stethoscope had become the badge of the progressive physician by 1820.

The London Medical Journal of 1827~1828, reported that there were those physicians who jumped on the stethoscopic bandwagon for the sake of appearances. One such, exuding an air of high professional competence, placed the wrong end of the stethoscope to his ear while holding the opposite end against the patient's chest. He gravely reported a respiratory murmur which turned out to be the rattle of a hackney coach passing on the street below.

In 1837, Oliver Wendell Holmes returned from his Paris studies and wrote a plea to his countrymen for the wider use of the stethoscope for direct exploration of the chest. By 1850 there were relatively few who were not using the monaural instrument routinely in office diagnosis.

There were many preferences for this new "mediate" auscultation. Some favored a solid turned cylinder, but most felt a hollow stethoscope allowed both wood and air to vibrate. Austin Flint, our most knowledgeable nineteenth century cardiologist, felt that wood did not conduct sound as well as metal or glass, but was lighter to use. He recommended the straight-fibered ebony and cedar. The latter, as well as pine, did not feel cold on the skin and were preferred by patients. These woods were less easily broken. Other woods included cherry or other fruitwood, mahogany and boxwood. Pewter, brass, silver, gutta percha and even papier mâché were fashioned into monaurals. Ivory was a handsome medium, but its poor sound conducting qualities relegated it to such as ear and chest pieces.

THE IDEAL MONAURAL

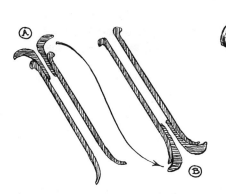

CHEST PIECE 1-1½" DIAMETER. ROUNDED EDGES FOR PATIENT COMFORT.

CONICAL HOLLOW.

6-9"

¼" BORE - CLEAR AND POLISHED.

½" STEM OF STRONG WOOD AS EBONY; 1" IF OF LIGHTER WOOD AS CEDAR.

EAR PIECE 2½" DIAMETER~ SHOULD COVER ENTIRE EAR AND BE VERY SLIGHTLY HOLLOWED. SOME SCREWED OR SLIPPED ON SHAFT, BUT A SINGLE PIECE OF TURNED WOOD WAS FELT SUPERIOR.

MANY STYLES AND SHAPES

GENERALLY, THE THICKER THE STEM, THE EARLIER THE PIECE. MANY OF THE EARLIEST EAR PIECES WERE IVORY. MOST METAL STETHOSCOPE APPEARED AFTER 1860.

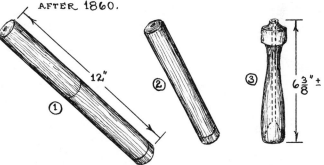

① 12"

②

③ 6⅜"±

1818-1819 LAENNEC ① + ②. HIS LAST IMPROVEMENT WAS ③~ A SHORTER, UNJOINTED TUBE WITH EARPIECE.

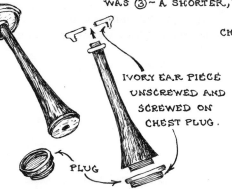

IVORY EAR PIECE UNSCREWED AND SCREWED ON CHEST PLUG.

PLUG

c.1828 DR. C.J.B. WILLIAMS, LONDON. THE EAR PIECE COULD BE REMOVED Ⓐ AND INSERTED INTO THE TRUMPET END Ⓑ AND THE VOICE EXAMINED WHILE LISTENING TO THE CHEST. FURTHER, THE STETHOSCOPE WAS MORE PORTABLE AND LESS EASILY DAMAGED WHEN CARRIED. OF SYCAMORE WOOD, IT WAS USED FOR "DELICATE SHADES OF SOUND."

1828 PIORRY ~ FRANCE. A HANDSOME STETHOSCOPE WITH IVORY FITTINGS WITH THE EAR PIECE SCREWED INTO THE PLUG. THE TRUMPET COULD SEE SERVICE AS A PLEXIMETER. (WELLCOME MUSEUM, LONDON)

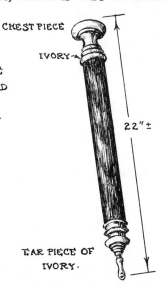

CHEST PIECE

IVORY

22"±

EAR PIECE OF IVORY.

c.1830 ENGLISH STETHOSCOPE PERHAPS INSPIRED BY LAENNEC'S, IT MUST HAVE BEEN LITTLE USED IN AMERICA. (WELLCOME MUSEUM, LONDON)

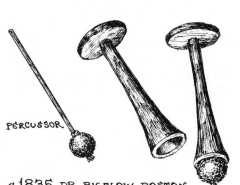

PERCUSSOR

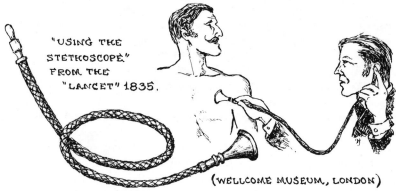

"USING THE STETHOSCOPE" FROM THE "LANCET" 1835.

(WELLCOME MUSEUM, LONDON)

c. 1835 DR. BIGELOW, BOSTON. ALL PURPOSE STETHOSCOPE. WIDE RIM OF EAR PIECE COULD BE USED AS A PLEXIMETER. THE PERCUSSOR, A WORSTED BALL COVERED WITH VELVET ON AN EBONY HANDLE, WAS CARRIED IN THE SOFT WOOD STETHOSCOPE.
(BOWDITCH 1846)

c. 1830~35 THE FLEXIBLE STETHOSCOPE. THIS NEW CONCEPT USED ONLY A COLUMN OF AIR AS THE CONDUCTING MEDIUM. CHEST SOUNDS WERE LOUD AND CLEAR AND WITHOUT MUCH OF ANY POSITIONAL CHANGE FROM THE PATIENT OR HIS PHYSICIAN.

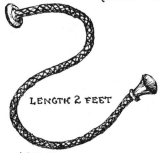

LENGTH 2 FEET

c. 1835 DR. PENNOCK'S, PHILADELPHIA. THE EAR AND CHEST WERE METAL. AS WITH THE 1830~35 MODEL, THE TUBE WAS COILED METALLIC WIRE COVERED WITH A SILK OR WORSTED WEB.
(BOWDITCH 1846)

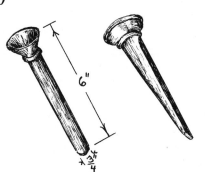

6"

3/4"

c. 1835~40 DRS. CAMMANN AND CLARK, U.S.A. SOLID SOFT WOOD STETHOSCOPE FOR AUSCULTORY PERCUSSION. THE WEDGE WAS USED BETWEEN THE RIBS.
(BOWDITCH 1846)

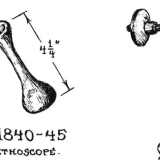

$4\frac{1}{4}$"

c. 1840~45 STETHOSCOPE. (WELLCOME MUSEUM)

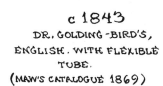

c 1843 DR. GOLDING-BIRD'S, ENGLISH. WITH FLEXIBLE TUBE. (MAW'S CATALOGUE 1869)

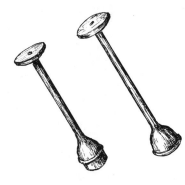

c. 1860 ~ SHORT AND LONG STETHOSCOPES. (MAW 1869)

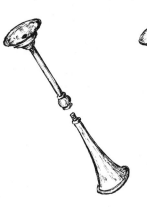

c. 1860 METAL TWO-PART STETHOSCOPE. (MAW 1869)

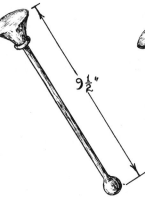

$9\frac{1}{2}$"

c. 1870~80 FETAL STETHOSCOPE OF SOLID WOOD. THE ROUNDED END WAS APPLIED TO THE MOTHER'S ABDOMEN. WELLCOME MUSEUM, LONDON)

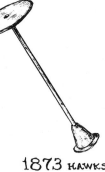

1873 HAWKSLEY'S. ONE OF MANY METAL VARIETIES OF THIS PERIOD. (TIEMANN CO. 1889)

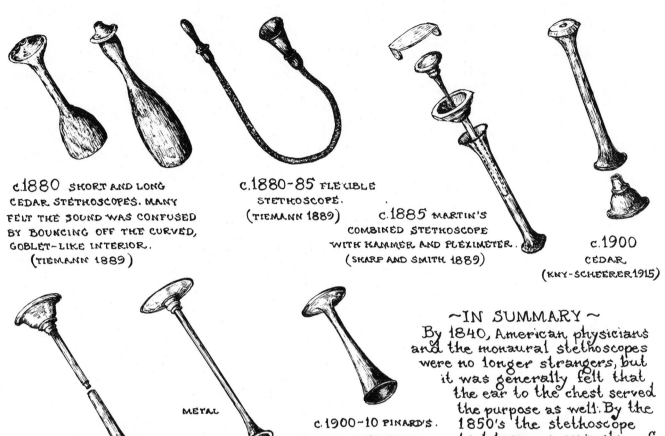

c.1880 SHORT AND LONG
CEDAR STETHOSCOPES. MANY
FELT THE SOUND WAS CONFUSED
BY BOUNCING OFF THE CURVED,
GOBLET-LIKE INTERIOR.
(TIEMANN 1889)

c.1880-85 FLEXIBLE
STETHOSCOPE.
(TIEMANN 1889)

c.1885 MARTIN'S
COMBINED STETHOSCOPE
WITH HAMMER AND PLEXIMETER.
(SHARP AND SMITH 1889)

c.1900
CEDAR.
(KNY-SCHEERER 1915)

METAL

c.1900-10 PINARD'S.
ALUMINUM FOR FETAL
HEART SOUNDS.
(KNY-SCHEERER 1915)

c.1900-05 TRAUBE'S.
TELESCOPIC METAL.
(KNY-SCHEERER 1915)

c.1900-05 HAWKSLEY'S.
TYPICAL OF LATE MONAURALS.
(KNY-SCHEERER 1915)

~IN SUMMARY~

By 1840, American physicians and the monaural stethoscopes were no longer strangers, but it was generally felt that the ear to the chest served the purpose as well. By the 1850's the stethoscope had become a mainstay of the physical examination. Countless styles and shapes were introduced in the last half of the nineteenth century, and most were advertized in the United States up to the First World War. But our physicians turned a deaf ear on the monaural in the 1860's when Cammann's binaural stethoscope made it obsolete.

THE BINAURAL STETHOSCOPE

As early as 1829, it had occurred to some that two ears were better than one. Several binaural efforts, however, gave only an awkward instrument with garbled sounds. It was in 1851 that Dr. Arthur Leared of Dublin presented his version at no less than the International Exposition in London. The two gutta-percha tubes, attached to the chest and ear pieces, made for a fairly workable stethoscope. Unfortunately, it caused little stir.

George Cammann of New York picked up the idea and ran with it. One year later he gave the world its first practical binaural stethoscope and a prototype for all those that would follow. Basically, the instrument was a marriage between a stubby monaural bell-shaped chest piece with two long air conduction tubes that were inspired by the flexible stethoscope.

Cammann's invention was no overnight success. His countrymen were not to be stampeded, particularly when the respected American authority Austin Flint gave a negative review in 1856. Fortunately, Flint reversed his views ten years later with the following enthusiastic endorsement for the Cammann binaural.

"After having now used it almost daily for more than ten years, I am much better prepared to speak of its merits. The objection on the score of the alteration of the pitch and quality of sounds I have long since found to be without foundation, and I am sure that this instrument will supplant all wooden stethoscopes as soon as it is fully appreciated. The power of conduction is greatly increased by the reception of the sounds simultaneously into both ears. Its superiority over instruments which conduct the sounds into one ear, is analogous to that of the binocular over the monocular microscope. The ease and comfort with which it is applied constitute not a small recommendation. The exclusion of other sounds than those conducted by the instrument is an important advantage. In short, to become so much attached to it as to dispense entirely with other stethoscopes, one need only to become accustomed to its use."

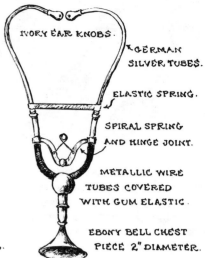

IVORY EAR KNOBS.

GERMAN SILVER TUBES.

ELASTIC SPRING.

SPIRAL SPRING AND HINGE JOINT.

METALLIC WIRE TUBES COVERED WITH GUM ELASTIC.

EBONY BELL CHEST PIECE 2" DIAMETER.

ORIGINAL 1852 CAMMANN BINAURAL.

By the late 1860's, most American physicians considered the Cammann binaural the standard for auscultory excellence. The old monaral was all but obsolete. Not so with their English counterparts, for it was not until the 1880's that they took any notice of the binaural stethoscope, and it was well into the twentieth century that its popularity lessened. Yet one of their countrymen made one of the early modifications to Cammann's invention. Scott Alison produced something of a double monaral stethoscope with not one but two chest bells ~ each with its own tube, one for each ear. His idea was to compare the sounds from different parts of the chest at the same time. This "differential" stethoscope captured considerable interest. Unfortunately, each ear received a weaker transmission than the usual binaural. Further, the listener found it difficult to compare different sounds when heard together and not separately ~ as with the notes of a musical instrument. It became a medical curiosity.

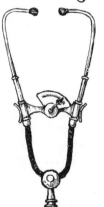

c.1860
ALISON'S DIFFERENTIAL
(DOWN BROS. 1889)

Many more Cammann modifications followed. The following have bell chest pieces.

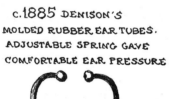

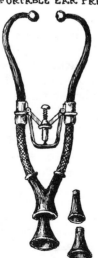

c.1880 PALMER'S.
A CIRCULAR BOX SPRING REPLACED THE ELASTIC BAND. USED AS A CALLIPER FOR MEASURING THE CHEST, HEAD, ETC.
(DOWN BROS. 1889)

c.1885 DENISON'S
MOLDED RUBBER EAR TUBES.
ADJUSTABLE SPRING GAVE COMFORTABLE EAR PRESSURE.

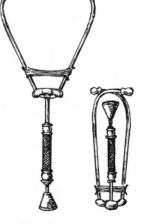

c.1885 GOWAN'S.
CONTINUOUS METAL CONDUCTION THROUGHOUT.
(DOWN BROS. 1889)

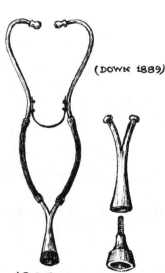

(DOWN 1889)

c.1885 FORD'S BELL.
SIMPLE, PORTABLE AND A WELL-DESERVED FAVORITE.

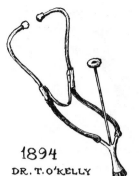

1894
DR. T. O'KELLY
(ENGLISH). THE 20 cm.
ROD AND RUBBER CUSHION
RESTED AGAINST THE FORE-
HEAD, LEAVING HANDS FREE
FOR PERCUSSION.
(DOWNS 1894)

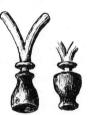

1896 SHEPPARD'S
FOLDING STETHOSCOPE.
(F.H.THOMAS 1918)

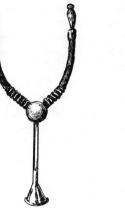

c.1900 SANSOM'S
OLD STYLE EAR PLUGS
(KNY-SCHEERER 1915)

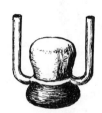

ENLARGED.

c.1900 OERTEL'S.
CONVERTABLE MONAURAL AND
BINAURAL — AND LOOKING MUCH LIKE
A MID-NINETEETH CENTURY VERSION!
(KNY-SCHEERER 1915)

Early twentieth century bell chest pieces with the Ford stethoscope.

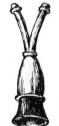

SNOFTON'S.
(BECTON-DICKSON 1917)

MEYER'S
WITH FINGER-REST.
(MORRIS)

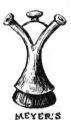

THOMPSON'S.
CHILDREN'S REVERSABLE.
(MORRIS)

ACME.
(F.H.THOMAS 1918)

GUY'S~WITH
ANTI-CHILL CUSHION
(MORRIS)

"DOME" MODEL WITH FIXED-SPRING
HEAD-FRAME. BASICALLY A BELL CHEST
PIECE WITH DIAPHRAGM-LIKE QUALITIES.
(MORRIS)

And later in the century~

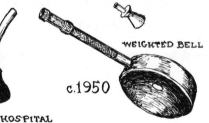

c.1927

WEIGHTED BELL

c.1950

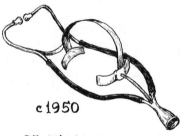

c.1950

ST. MARY'S HOSPITAL
(MORRIS)

LEFF FOETAL STETHOSCOPE (MORRIS)

DE LEE HILLIS FOETAL STETHOSCOPE (MORRIS)

The Cammann binaural had made its mark on the medical world. And so it was in America until one of its many modifications, the Ford model, become the standard for bell chest piece auscultation. Early on, the bells were of turned wood, ivory, metal, and even ceramic. The mid-Victorians early plastic, gutta-percha, was incorporated in both the Leared and Denison's binaurals. The dried sap from a Borneo tree, Dichopsis gutta, could be heated and molded into the intricate stethoscope parts. Hard rubber discs were frequent insertions into later metal bell chest pieces. Soft rubber anti-chill coverings gave patient comfort since James Murray had the idea in 1889.

THE DIAPHRAGM CHEST PIECE

The bell chest piece was invaluable for producing pure heart sounds, particularly those in the lower frequency range. It also gave good service when localizing foetal heart sounds and those of the lung. Yet there were high frequency sounds that could be missed. Enter the diaphragm chest piece with its membrane that could vibrate much like the human ear drum. Then those illusive soft, high-pitched murmurs and like sounds could help piece together the physical diagnosis.

The initial diaphragm efforts were less than inspiring. Dr. Alison, of differential stethoscope fame, came forth with his "hydrophone" in 1861. Listening to a thin and bony individual with the bell chest piece had been something of a problem. The sunken intercostal spaces defied stethoscope contact until this water-filled rubber bag~ about the size of a large pocket watch~ filled the spaces nicely. Unfortunately, the bag somewhat muffled the sounds that struggled through to the stethoscope.

A promising diaphragm model was suggested by Dr. Charles Hogeboin of New York City. He stretched a piece of parchment under tension over a Cammann bell chest piece. When placed against the chest, according to our early authority Austin Flint, "the power of conduction seems to me to be increased without other change, and the source of the sounds appears to be circumscribed by the addition of the parchment."

Perhaps inspired by this early trial, a host of outlandish diaphragm stethoscopes hit the medical market in the last quarter of the nineteenth century. Many were cleverly conceived while others were downright Rube Goldburgish.

They made their debute under such high-sounding names as hydrophones, phonophores, phonendoscopes, stethonoscopes and ampli-phones.

A more practical chest piece was transitional between the bell and the diaphragm. Dr. Kehler's 1897 version had a wide-rimmed bell disc~ and a novel swivel arrangement that allowed for slipping the piece under clothing. A somewhat similar Yale stethoscope was patented in 1906.

c.1887

AMPLIPHONE WITH RESONATING METAL DIAPHRAGMS AND A BELL FOR EXACT SOUND LOCATION.
(F.C. THOMAS 1918)

PHONENDOSCOPE APART.
1894

COMPACTED PHONENDOSCOPE.
BAZZI & BIANCHI'S, 2½" DIAMETER.
DETACKABLE LOCALIZER, AND WOUND TUBING WITH VULCANITE EAR PIECES.
(ALLEN & HANBURY 1930)

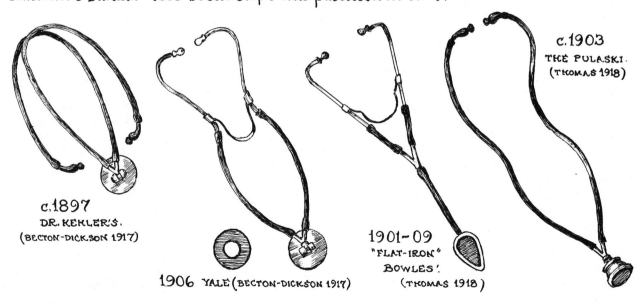

c.1897
DR. KEHLER'S.
(BECTON-DICKSON 1917)

1906 YALE (BECTON-DICKSON 1917)

1901~09
"FLAT-IRON" BOWLES.
(THOMAS 1918)

c.1903
THE PULASKI.
(THOMAS 1918)

The standard for all subsequent "resonating stethoscopes" was the Bowles' diaphragm chest piece of 1898. At first of a flat-iron shape before the familiar disc version, it was connected to the Cammann binaural style tubes with a flat steel spring. This simple and efficient diaphragm took its place beside the Ford bell for a more complete auscultation in American physical examinations.

COMBINATION STETHOSCOPES

It was inevitable that the Ford bell and the Bowles' diaphragm became a diagnostic team. Robert Bowles of Boston patented the first combination chest piece in 1902. His original diaphragm disc was connected to a short tube that could be plugged into a bell. But it was a marriage that had its awkward separations. Then Dr. Howard Sprague of that same city called on his Yankee ingenuity, and by 1926 had invented the first really efficient bell and diaphragm unit. With a flick of a lever the conversion could be made — and without the bothersome detachments of Bowles' earlier model. It was immediately popular, and still may be purchased as its Rieger-Bowles model.

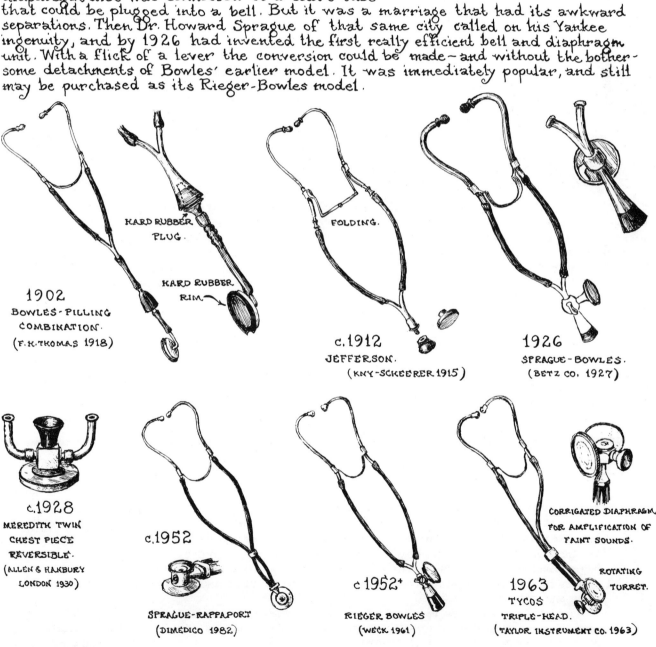

(MUTTER MUSEUM)

1937
KERR SYMBALLOPHONE, REMINISCENT OF THE OLD ALISON'S DIFFERENTIAL BELL STETHOSCOPE. SOUNDS FROM DIFFERENT POINTS COULD BE COMPARED.

HARD RUBBER PLUG.

HARD RUBBER RIM

1902
BOWLES-PILLING COMBINATION.
(F.H. THOMAS 1918)

FOLDING.

c.1912
JEFFERSON.
(KNY-SCHEERER 1915)

1926
SPRAGUE-BOWLES.
(BETZ CO. 1927)

c.1928
MEREDITH TWIN CHEST PIECE REVERSIBLE.
(ALLEN & HANBURY LONDON 1930)

c.1952
SPRAGUE-RAPPAPORT
(DIMEDICO 1982)

c.1952+
RIEGER BOWLES
(WECK 1961)

CORRIGATED DIAPHRAGM FOR AMPLIFICATION OF FAINT SOUNDS.

ROTATING TURRET.

1963
TYCOS TRIPLE-HEAD.
(TAYLOR INSTRUMENT CO. 1963)

1961 LITTMANN.

The Sprague Bowles model inspired other spin-offs, including the Sprague-Rappaport with its interchangeable three bell and two diaphragm chest pieces, the weighty Tycos triple change (9½ oz) with a bell and two diaphragms, and the English version (Meredith). All revolved on a stem for positioning.

With a wide range and variety of sounds available, increasing the loudness was obviously desirable. Since the air in the hollow binaural tubing transmitted the intensity of sound inversely as the volume of air, efforts were made to decrease the bore diameter. Dr. David Littmann of Boston brought forth an admirable instrument that contained an extremely small amount of air in its Tygan tubing. The sounds were loud and clear from its reversable chest pieces. Light (2 oz) and easily carried, the stethoscope is the all-American favorite as of this writing!

ELECTRIC STETHOSCOPES

There was another way to increase sound intensity - electricity. The two examples of electrical sound amplifiers span much of our twentieth century.

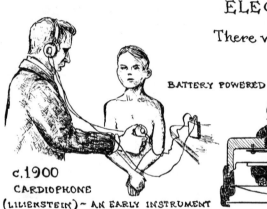

BATTERY POWERED

c.1900
CARDIOPHONE
(LILIENSTEIN) ~ AN EARLY INSTRUMENT
FOR MAGNIFYING HEART SOUNDS ELECTRICALLY
(KNY-SCHEERER 1915)

1982
ELECTRONIC STETHOSCOPE. ALL ELECTRONICS ARE IN THE CHEST PIECE AND THE AMPLIFIER SELF CONTAINED IN THE TUBING. ALL MINIA-TURIZED SOLID STATE AMPLIFICATION TO 100 TIMES. OPERATES ON 2 HEARING AID BATTERIES.   (SCHEIN CO. 1982)

~IN SUMMARY~

MONAURAL STETHOSCOPES ~ Elastic (fibrous), straight-grained less dense woods, as ebony and cedar, increased the intensity of vibrations. When the stem bulk was reduced by the mid-nineteenth century, the intensity of sound was further increased. Solid wood stethoscopes were used to auscultate solid body masses such as the heart or foetal heart. However, surface friction noises competed with internal sounds. By boring a central hole, the transmission of sounds through the air added sounds not otherwise heard. The shorter the air column and the smaller the bore diameter the better.

THE CHEST PIECE SHOULD BE TWO INCHES OR LESS FOR BETTER LOCALIZATION. THE EAR PIECES SHOULD BE 2½ INCHES TO FIT THE EAR CLOSELY TO PREVENT DISPERSIONS OF THE VIBRATIONS.

BINAURAL ~ The tubing was of India rubber. Today, it is of latex or silicone rubber. It should be thick, about ten inches long, and fit the connections snugly. The internal calibre, including the metal ear tubes and the hole in the center of the chest piece, should be one eighth of an inch in diameter.

THE BELL CUP SHOULD BE RATHER SHALLOW WITH A DIAMETER NOT LESS THAN AN INCH. ITS LOW PITCHED SOUNDS ARE ACCENTUATED BY LIGHT CHEST PRESSURE. FIRM CHEST PRESSURE GIVES HIGHER PITCHED SOUNDS.

THE BOWLES SHOULD BE 1½ INCHES IN DIAMETER WITH A SHALLOW CUP AND AN ANTI-CHILL RIM OF RUBBER OR PLASTIC. THE DIAPHRAGM OF X-RAY FILM TRANSMITS HIGH PITCHED SOUNDS.

BELL.

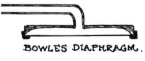

BOWLES DIAPHRAGM.

BLOOD PRESSURE INSTRUMENTS

BLOOD PRESSURE IS THAT PRESSURE OF THE BLOOD WITHIN THE ARTERIES, PRIMARILY MAINTAINED BY THE CONTRACTION OF THE LEFT VENTRICLE. THE SYSTOLIC PRESSURE IS THE HIGHEST PRESSURE DURING ONE CARDIAC CYCLE AT THE MOMENT THE CREST OF THE PULSE WAVE ARRIVES. THE DIASTOLIC PRESSURE IS THE LOWEST PRESSURE OF THAT CYCLE.

Back in 1806, Thomas Jefferson wrote to Edward Jenner that "Harvey's discovery of the circulation of the blood was a beautiful addition to our knowledge of animal economy, but on a review of the practice of medicine before and since that epoch, I do not see any great amelioration which has been derived from that discovery." Jefferson was, of course, referring to William Harvey's declaration in 1628 that "a perpetual movement of blood in a circle is caused by the beat of the heart."

The force required of this human pump to push blood through its closed elastic plumbing system varied with health and disease. Our earliest American physicians could make a guesstimate of this pressure by palpating a "hard" or "soft" pulse, or by applying a steady finger pressure on the artery until the pulse disappeared. Obviously, the higher the blood pressure, the greater the finger pressure necessary to occlude it.

But Jefferson was right. Each practitioner had his own interpretation of what he felt. There was no standard – no measurement – that could be compared or reproduced.

There were early efforts to solve the problem. An English minister, Stephen Hales, made the first attempt by inserting a nine-foot glass tube directly into the femoral artery of a cooperative horse. Then, in 1828, the French physiologist Léonard Poiseille followed up on the idea with mercury in a bent glass tube to counterbalance the pressure of the blood. The lengthy tube of Hales was no longer needed, but the normals for the height of mercury were yet to be solved.

Karl Ludwig continued this experimental work on animals with a mercury float and an attached pen. A paper-wrapped revolving drum recorded the pressure variations. With any sort of standard lacking, no patient was about to consent to having his artery invaded and see his life's blood run through the tubing!

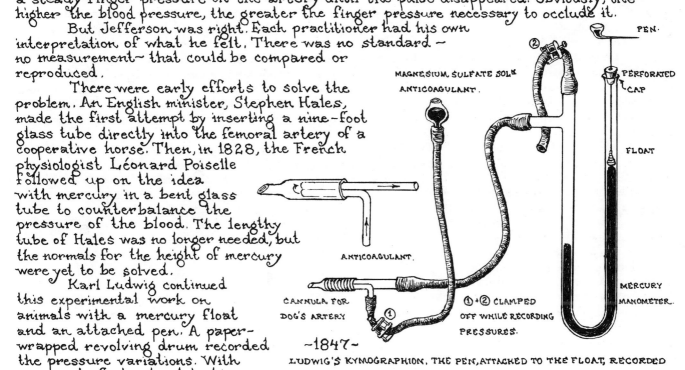

MAGNESIUM SULFATE SOLᴺ ANTICOAGULANT.

PEN.

PERFORATED CAP

FLOAT

ANTICOAGULANT.

CANNULA FOR DOG'S ARTERY

① + ② CLAMPED OFF WHILE RECORDING PRESSURES.

MERCURY MANOMETER.

~1847~
LUDWIG'S KYMOGRAPHION, THE PEN, ATTACHED TO THE FLOAT, RECORDED THE ARTERIAL PRESSURE FLUCTUATIONS ON THE REVOLVING DRUM.

All the preceeding experimental work on animals climaxed in 1860 when the first clinically useful pulse and pressure recorder was invented. The credit for the new sphygmograph belonged to the French physician Etienne-Jules Marey. Its lever rested on the artery – not in it – while the other end scratched the undulations onto a strip of smoked paper. This moved at a uniform rate, thanks to a clockwork mechanism at its base. Interpreting the data was another matter, and the device was more practical for research than in the doctor's office. Still and all, it was a long stride forward in the

1857
MAREY'S WRIST SPHYGMOGRAPH.

search for a convenient, simplified measure of the patient's circulation.

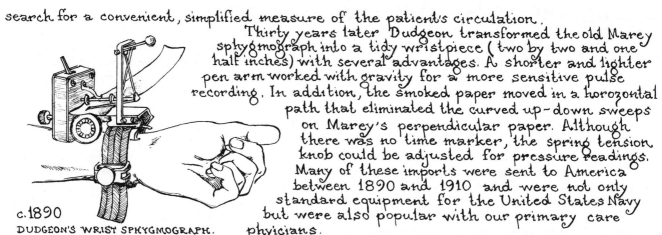

Thirty years later Dudgeon transformed the old Marey sphygmograph into a tidy wristpiece (two by two and one half inches) with several advantages. A shorter and lighter pen arm worked with gravity for a more sensitive pulse recording. In addition, the smoked paper moved in a horizontal path that eliminated the curved up-down sweeps on Marey's perpendicular paper. Although there was no time marker, the spring tension knob could be adjusted for pressure readings. Many of these imports were sent to America between 1890 and 1910 and were not only standard equipment for the United States Navy but were also popular with our primary care phyicians.

c.1890
DUDGEON'S WRIST SPHYGMOGRAPH.

There were more to follow. In 1890, Jacquet's Original Sphygmocardiograph added an interval timer to more accurately record rate and rhythm. The 1910 "Improved" model produced more accurate vibration frequency recordings. Also that year Jacquet's "Transmission Sphygmograph" contained an innovative five speed clock that could highlight irregular beats by slowing down the pulse recording.

In 1902 Mackenzie's Portable Polygraph used ink to do away with the messy smoked paper, and contained a clock that could regulate the recording speed. And, by 1920, the Sanborn Polygraph had incorporated most of the desirable features of its predecessors to make it more sturdy, compact and trouble free. But almost before its introduction, the new sphygmomanometers were moving the sphymograph concept into the backwaters of history.

THE SPHYGMOMETER ("Sphygmo~" = pulse)

The rise and fall of the sphygmograph featured these ingenious little machines that seemed more useful for laboratory research than in a clinical setting. Still, they did stimulate considerable interest in the importance of the pulse and blood pressure in physical diagnosis.

The sphygmometer approached the problem from a different angle. Since the blood pressure within an artery was equal to the force necessary to collapse the vessel, it seemed reasonable that this force might be measured. The sphygmometer supplied the force— as well as the blood pressure reading when the pulse below it ceased. To be effective, the artery must be pressed against an overlying bone.

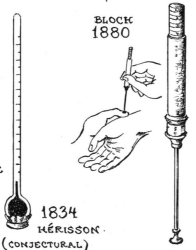

BLOCK
1880

1834
HÉRISSON
(CONJECTURAL)

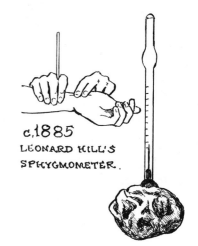

c.1885
LEONARD HILL'S
SPHYGMOMETER.

Jules Hérisson had the idea in 1834 when physicians could only estimate the blood pressure by palpation. His original sphygmometer was a straight glass calibrated tube that ended with a cuplike base. Over its mouth was stretched a skin membrane. When filled with mercury, the membrane was pressed over the radial artery. Unfortunately, it was difficult to steady the cup and to apply the pressure necessary to give any sort of accuracy.

Block's instrument of 1880 applied force on the palpating finger, which in turn felt for the obliteration of the pulse. The pressure was then read from the sliding barrel markings. Five years later, Cheron improved the instrument to the extent that a plunger foot compressed the artery alone. The barrel pressure markings were recorded when the pulse below the plunger disappeared.

Hill's Pocket Sphygmometer returned to the measured column of mercury with the addition of a rubber bulb. This was pressed on the radial artery and the pressure read when its peripheral pulse was obliterated. Problems included considerable variation in the readings and no way to determine the diastolic pressure. In short, the sphygmometers' claim to fame was its portability.

THE SPHYGMOMANOMETER

The first real breakthrough in the search for a clinically workable blood pressure instrument came in 1876. Vienna's Professor Samuel von Basch earned his place in medical history with his experimental sphygmomanometer. The manometer was a calibrated "U" tube with a pinch cock that could be opened to level the mercury at zero. A glass cup, faced with a loosely stretched elastic membrane, was filled with water, as was the connecting manometer tubing. With one hand, the physician gradually pressed the cup against the patient's radial or temporal arteries, while the other hand felt the diminishing pulse. When no further pulse was felt, the pressure was read from the scale in millimeters of mercury. Although the instrument never reached the assembly line, its accuracy inspired the many that would follow.

Von Basch's invention gave birth to several impressive offspring. Von Basch's Portable, c.1880, and Potain's sphygmomanometer of 1889, substituted a spring clock manometer with von Basch's arterial compression balloon and tubal connections containing water and air respectively. Both were near misses, but their spring clock manometer concept developed into a long line of aneroid drums along the lines of the atmospheric barometer. (More on this important group later.)

1876
VON BASCH
(REICHERT COLLECTION)

Meanwhile, Riva-Ricci's sphygmomanometer of 1895 carried on the mercury monometer tradition of von Basch with a single tube and a base reservoir, instead of the "U" tube. More important was complete compression of the artery with 360° of pressure from a rubber bag that encircled the arm. Anatomical variations of the artery's location, as well as slippage and the lack of uniform pressure from the von Basch's cup membrane (pelotte) were no longer a problem.

When air was pumped in, the systolic pressure was read on the mercury

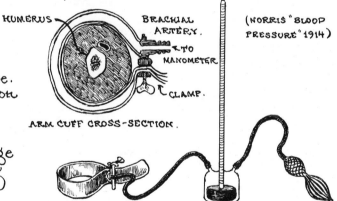

ARM CUFF CROSS-SECTION.

(NORRIS "BLOOD PRESSURE" 1914)

1895 RIVA-ROCCI'S SPHYGMOMANOMETER.

column when the palpating fingers below the cuff felt the pulse disappear. And finally, the diastolic pressure could also be taken – a real advance toward diagnosing the hypertensive patient. The release valve on the cuff was opened, and the pulse beat followed down until no longer felt. This was the lower reading – the diastolic pressure. All this should have a familiar ring to it – his instrument has the basic features of those in use today.

Before 1900 it was a rare physician who would tolerate the inconveniences and inaccuracies of reading a blood pressure. Riva-Rocci had made such a measurement practical. By 1910, a majority of American physicians were using this diagnostic device with enthusiasm. American instrument makers were quick to appreciate the demand, and new advances in design created many new models in the years ahead.

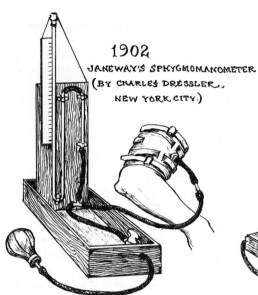

1902
JANEWAY'S SPHYGMOMANOMETER
(BY CHARLES DRESSLER,
NEW YORK CITY.)

1903
H.W. COOK'S SPHYGMOMANOMETER
(BY ELMER & AMEND, NEW YORK CITY.)
A MODIFICATION OF RIVA-ROCCI.

1905
H.W. COOK'S PORTABLE.

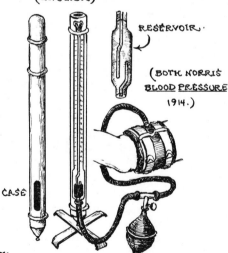

AN EARLY AMERICAN FAVORITE AND WAS
FIRST TO HAVE A CARRYING BOX. THE
"U" TUBE OF VON BASCH WAS MORE EASILY
CALIBRATED, AND THE WIDER CUFF ($4\frac{5}{8}$")
GAVE BETTER COMPRESSION. THE SCALE
SLID DOWN INTO THE BOX WHEN NOT IN
USE. ACCURATE, LIGHT AND COMPACT, ITS
RUBBER JOINTS WERE FRAIL AND THE
MERCURY EASILY SPILLED WHEN NOT USED.
(NORRIS BLOOD PRESSURE, 1914)

AMERICA'S VERSION OF
THE RIVA ROCCI'S INSTRUMENT
(TAUGHT BLOOD PRESSURE 1913)
THE PORTABLE VERSION HAD A JOINTED MANOMETER
TUBE FOR EASIER PACKING. TO PREVENT LEAKAGE WHEN
BOXED, CORKS WERE INSERTED INTO THE TIP OF THE MERCURY
TUBE AND ITS OUTLET AND THE BASE RESERVOIR CONTAINED
A TRAP. IN SPITE OF BEING SECURED TO THE BASE, THE
MANOMETER, UNFORTUNATELY, WAS EASILY UPSET AND BROKEN.
CALIBRATION WAS DIFFICULT AND THE NARROW CUFF GAVE
EXCESSIVELY HIGH READINGS.   (KNY-SCHEERER 1915)

In 1905, Korotkow
suggested that the blood pressure should be taken by auscultation with a stethoscope
below the cuff instead of palpation. Its simplicity and accuracy quickly doomed the
earlier technique.

c.1910 DR. OLIVER'S PORTABLE
COMPRESSED AIR MANOMETER.

1910 LEONARD HILL SPHYGMOMANOMETER
(ENGLISH)

1911 MERCER
DRESSER-BEARD MFG.CO., N.Y.

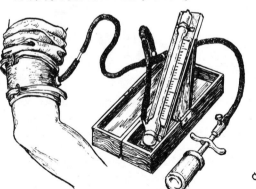

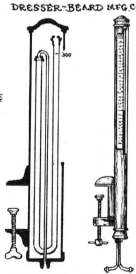

RESERVOIR
(BOTH NORRIS
BLOOD PRESSURE
1914.)

CASE

(HAWKSLEY & SONS, LONDON, ENGLAND.)
THE SEALED END OF THE MANOMETER
TRAPPED AIR ABOVE THE MERCURY COLUMN, THEREBY
SHORTENING THE TUBE TO ONE FOURTH THE
USUAL LENGTH. HOWEVER, TEMPERATURE WOULD
EXPAND THE AIR TO GIVE FALSE READINGS. VERY
PORTABLE WITH THE CUFF AND PUMP CARRIED
SEPARATELY, IT WAS MORE POPULAR IN
ENGLAND AND FRANCE (NORRIS 1914)

THIS RIVA-ROCCI TYPE HAD A
TINY BORE THAT PREVENTED ANY
MERCURY SPILLAGE. IT WAS VERY
PORTABLE IN ITS WOODEN CASE,
ALTHOUGH THE CUFF AND PUMP
WERE CARRIED SEPARATELY. ACCURATE.

"U" TYPE ENTIRELY ENCLOSED
BY A METAL HOUSING AND HELD
IN PLACE BY MELTED WAX. A
TABLE CLAMP SECURED THIS
PORTABLE INSTRUMENT. THE
SMALL SCALE WAS HARD TO READ.

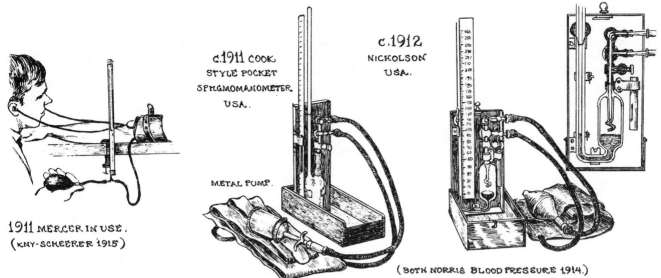

1911 MERCER IN USE.
(KNY-SCHEERER 1915)

c.1911 COOK
STYLE POCKET
SPHYGMOMANOMETER.
USA.

METAL PUMP.

c.1912
NICKOLSON
USA.

(BOTH NORRIS BLOOD PRESSURE 1914.)

THE POPULARITY OF ACCURATE SPHYGMOMANOMETERS WAS SKYROCKETING, AND AMERICA'S INSTRUMENT MAKERS PULLED OUT ALL THE STOPS TO PRODUCE AN ACCURATE, STURDY, SIMPLE AND PORTABLE PRODUCT. THE NEW COOK STYLE WAS QUICKLY REPLACED BY THE NICKOLSON. THE MERCURY WAS LEVELED TO "0" WITH A STOPCOCK — ACCURATE REGARDLESS OF TEMPERATURE CHANGES. A LARGE COLUMN OF MERCURY PREVENTED ITS SEPARATION AS WELL AS OXIDATION AND CAPILLARY ERRORS. A SPECIAL STOPCOCK GUARRANTEED NO MERCURY LEAKAGE. BOTH USE THE MORE EFFICIENT $4\frac{1}{2}$ INCH WIDE CUFF.

In 1901, von Recklinghausen had shown that a cuff of four and one half inches in width gave proper arterial compression. The narrow cuff needed additional pressure to indent the tissues and vessels and therefore gave excessively high readings. Too wide a cuff gave low readings with insufficient pressure on the tissues and vessel. By 1910, most of the sphygmomanometers conformed to his standard.

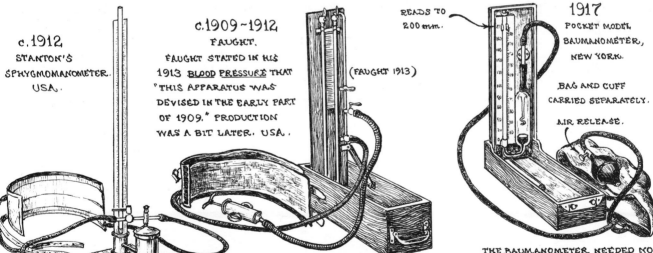

c.1912
STANTON'S
SPHYGMOMANOMETER.
USA.

c.1909~1912
FAUGHT.
FAUGHT STATED IN HIS
1913 BLOOD PRESSURE THAT
"THIS APPARATUS WAS
DEVISED IN THE EARLY PART
OF 1909." PRODUCTION
WAS A BIT LATER. USA.

(FAUGHT 1913)

READS TO
200 mm.

1917
POCKET MODEL
BAUMANOMETER,
NEW YORK.

BAG AND CUFF
CARRIED SEPARATELY.

AIR RELEASE.

CHANGES INCLUDED A METAL CISTERN, AND A STOPCOCK LEADING TO THE INFLATING BULB TO LESSEN ITS ELASTICITY DURING THE DIASTOLIC READING. HOWEVER, THE CISTERN GAVE LOW READINGS WITH HIGH PRESSURES, AND TIME AND MERCURY WERE LOST IN THE SETTING-UP PROCESS. (FAUGHT 1913)

GUARD COCKS ARE ON EACH "U" TUBE ARM TO PREVENT MERCURY LOSS BUT MUST BE OPENED WHEN IN USE. THE UPPER STOPCOCK TO THE PUMP MUST BE CLOSED FOR SYSTOLIC AND DIASTOLIC READINGS. A COLLAPSIBLE RUBBER PUMP TUBE REDUCED THE IMPACT OF AIR AND NO SECOND BULB IS NECESSARY. RUGGED AND ACCURATE.

THE BAUMANOMETER NEEDED NO ADJUSTMENTS. THE LARGE BORE TUBE PREVENTED THE OXIDATION OF MERCURY AND AIR POCKETS. A SIMPLE ONE-PIECE TUBE REQUIRED NO LEAKY VALVES AS WITH THE OLDER MULTIPLE CONNECTIONS. THE EASILY READ SCALE WAS ACCURATE. THE COMPACT BOX (10" X 3" X 1½") WAS EASILY CARRIED. THIS PROTOTYPE WAS IMMEDIATELY POPULAR.

1919 BAUMANOMETER
THIS IMPROVED INSTRUMENT LOOKED MUCH LIKE ITS PREDECESSOR BUT HAD A SLIGHTLY LONGER TUBE AND WIDER RESERVOIR. THIS GAVE A LARGER SCALE THAT READ TO 260mm.

c.1921 BAUMANOMETER, WALL-BOARD MODEL.

c.1921 BAUMANOMETER, DESK MODEL.

c.1926 BECTON DICKINSON
THE METAL CAP WAS FITTED WITH A METAL GAUZE DISC AND SPECIAL METAL DISC TO ALLOW AIR PASSAGE BUT TO HOLD MERCURY IN.

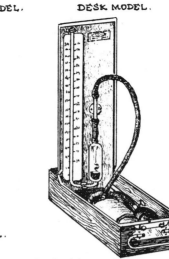

16" X 6" X ¾"
SCALE TO 300 mm.

(BAUM CO., N.Y.— N.D.)

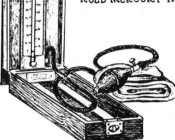

THE 1924~26 MODEL ENCLOSED THE RESERVOIR IN A METAL CONTAINER.

(BETZCO 1927)

c.1926 BECTON-DICKINSON POCKET MANOMETER.

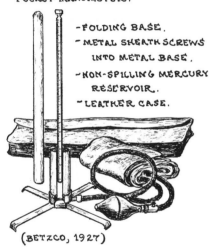

- FOLDING BASE.
- METAL SHEATH SCREWS INTO METAL BASE.
- NON-SPILLING MERCURY RESERVOIR.
- LEATHER CASE.

(BETZCO, 1927)

The 1917~1921 Baumanometer classics and the later Becton-Dickinson variation are basically unchanged to the present day. Reliability and accuracy remain hallmarks, but old timers must miss those handsomely polished walnut cases that were replaced by metal containers.

CLOCK~TYPE SPHYGMOMANOMETERS

A late bloomer on the arterial blood pressure scene was the clock style sphygmomanometer. Although never popular in America, they did pave the way for the less finicky aneroid instruments. The heart of the clock manometer was the Bourdon spring - a hollow, curved, thin metal tube that was sealed at one end. When water or air was pumped in under pressure, the hollow tube tended to straighten. This in turn moved a hair spring and its needle indicator. The Bourdon spring group included:

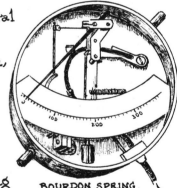

BOURDON SPRING.

c.1887 VON BASCH'S.

1889 POTAIN'S.

1908 VON RECKLINGHAUSEN.

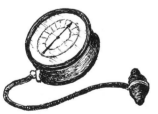

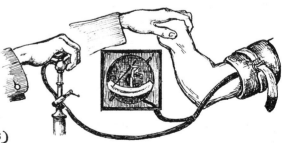

(WELLCOME MUSEUM, LONDON)
WATER WAS USED IN THE COMPRESSION SYSTEM.
THE BULB (PELOTTE) OBLITERATED THE ARTERY BY FINGER PRESSURE. OFTEN MORE PRESSURE WAS APPLIED TO THE SURROUNDING TISSUES THAN THE ARTERY ITSELF.

(KNY-SCHEERER CATALOGUE 1915)
AIR REPLACED THE WATER OF VON BASCH'S.

THE BICYCLE PUMP INFLATED THE CUFF AND THE HOLLOW BOURDON SPRING. MORE ACCURATE THAN ITS PREDECESSORS.

ANEROID SPHGMOMANOMETERS (Aneroid = dry)

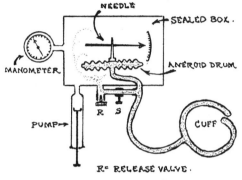

CHAIN — POINTER — MAINSPRING
AXLE — VACUUM BOX
ANEROID BAROMETER.

American physicians had been less than enthusiastic over the cumbersome and inaccurate turn-of-the-century mercurial sphygmomanometer. The Bourdon spring principle had its possibilities and its problems—enough to consider it something of medical curiosity on this side of the Atlantic. But there was yet another method of measuring pressure—atmospheric pressure, that is. The well-known aneroid barometer was an airtight vacuum box that responded to changes in the air.

In 1909, Pachon adapted this principle in reverse by enclosing a thin metal drum in a sealed box, free from any atmospheric variations. The pressure inside the aneroid drum was equal to that on its outer surface, making the connected cuff and its pulse transmissions all the more sensitive and accurate.

NEEDLE — SEALED BOX.
MANOMETER — ANEROID DRUM
PUMP — CUFF
R S
R = RELEASE VALVE.
S = SEPARATING BUTTON.
PACHON'S DIAGRAM.

Briefly, the pump gave uniform pressure in the box, cuff and aneroid drum. The pump pressure was first increased above the artery's systolic pressure. The release valve was opened briefly to slightly lower the overall pressure as indicated on the manometer. Then the separator button closed off the box pressure, thereby isolated the air in the cuff and the drum. A series of such manipulations continued until the first pulse pressure oscillations were seen in the drum needle. This was the systolic pressure and was recorded from the manometer. The pressure reduction alternated with the separating button closure until the greatest needle oscillations were produced. This was the diastolic pressure and was read from the manometer. However, these accurate recordings were time-consuming and hardly a simple procedure in the average physician's office.

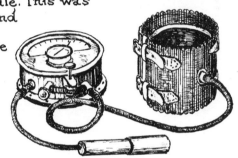

The aneroid idea caught fire. The Tag Roesch sphygmomanometer was introduced about a year after Pachon's invention— and it had real promise. Several aneroid drums moved under pressure in progressively smaller excursions to prevent distortion of the metal and to insure accuracy. Reichert states that "this anaeroid drum series is used in almost all of the better American instruments since approximately 1910."

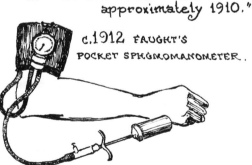

ANEROID DIAGRAM.

c.1912 FAUGHT'S POCKET SPHGMOMANOMETER.

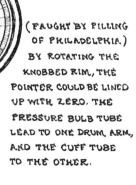

(FAUGHT BY PILLING OF PHILADELPHIA) BY ROTATING THE KNOBBED RIM, THE POINTER COULD BE LINED UP WITH ZERO. THE PRESSURE BULB TUBE LEAD TO ONE DRUM ARM, AND THE CUFF TUBE TO THE OTHER.

Dr. Rogers instrument of 1913 contained four aneroid drums in series. It and the 1915 and 1917 models promptly became the most popular aneroid sphygmomanometer in America. There were many similarities to the Faught model.

The continued excellence of the mercurial Baumanometers these many years was paralleled in the anaeroid field by the Tycos sphygmomanometer. For almost thirty years, the "Dr. Rogers" trademark saw service in increasing numbers. The man behind the name was its inventor, Dr. Oscar H. Rogers, medical director of the New York Life Insurance Company. The company behind the man was Taylor Instrument of Rochester, New York.

1907~14
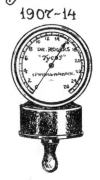

DR. ROGERS-TYCOS.
(KNY-SCHEERER 1915)

1915~26
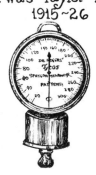

DR. ROGERS-TYCOS.
(TAYLOR INSTRUMENT ADV. 1916)

1927~31+
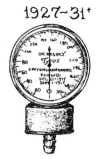

DR. ROGERS-TYCOS.
(TAYLOR INSTRUMENT ADV. 1927)

THE "DR. ROGERS" TRADEMARK CONTINUED UNTIL THE EARLY 1930's. WITH ITS "SELF-VERIFYING" 1915 FEATURE, INSTRUMENT ACCURACY WAS GUARANTEED IF THE POINTER RESTED INSIDE THE OVAL "ZERO". THOSE TYCOS MODELS THAT FOLLOWED CONTINUED TO EMPHASIZE THIS AS WELL AS IT BEING A COMPACT AND LIGHT POCKET AND BEDSIDE INSTRUMENT.

MINOR FACIAL CHANGES HELP TO DETERMINE "DR. ROGERS'" AGE. THE 1907-1914 SCALE READ TO 26 mm. WITH NO PATENT NOTATION. 1915~1926 READ TO 300 mm. ALONG WITH THE INSCRIPTION "PAT. PEND." THE 1927 MODEL AND THEREAFTER ALSO READ TO 300 mm., BUT HAD "PATENTED DEC. 21-1915 SEPT. 1-1917. THOSE EARLIER DATES ON A LATER INSTRUMENT HAVE CREATED SOME CONFUSION AMONG ANTIQUE MEDICAL INSTRUMENT COLLECTORS.

1925
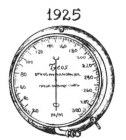

OFFICE STYLE-TYCOS.
6" DIAL. WIRE EASEL FOR TABLE OR FASTENED TO WALL.
(SHARP & SMITH 1925)

1937
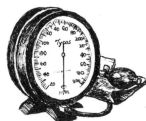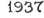

DESK MODEL-TYCOS.
(TAYLOR INSTRUMENT ADV. 1937)

1956
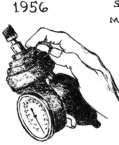

HAND MODEL-TYCOS.
INFLATING BULB AND AIR RELEASE VALVE ARE BUILT INTO THE BACK OF THE GUAGE.
(TAYLOR INSTRUMENT ADV. 1956)

1961
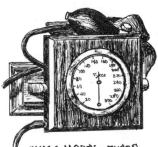

WALL MODEL-TYCOS.
(WECK & CO. 1961)

1963
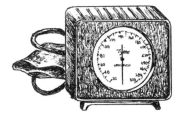

DESK ANEROID-TYCOS.
(TAYLOR INSTRUMENT ADV 1963)

1982
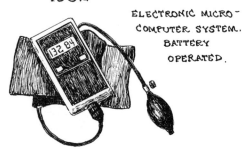

ELECTRONIC MICRO-COMPUTER SYSTEM. BATTERY OPERATED.

ACOUSTIC SPHYGMOMANOMETER.

IN 1946, THE CUMBERSOME LONG-TAILED "WRAP-AROUND CUFF GAVE WAY TO THE HOOK-CUFF. IT WAS 5 TIMES FASTER TO HOOK A METAL BUTTON INTO A STAINLESS STEEL RIB.

1946
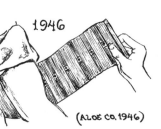

(ALOE CO. 1946)

1963

THEN THE HOOK-CUFF LOST OUT TO THE VELCRO CUFF FASTENER. PRESS ON AND PEEL OFF IN A MOMENT, AND THE TINY HOOKS AND OPPOSITE LOOPS SNAGGED EACH OTHER SECURELY.

ELECTROCARDIOGRAPHS

In 1794, the Professor of Anatomy at the University of Bologna stumbled upon one of the body's deepest secrets. Aloysio Galvani observed that the partially dissected legs of a frog contracted whenever a nearby electrostatic machine was rotated. A metal scalpel had been left in contact with an exposed nerve. Further experiments convinced Galvani that electricity was actually produced in living tissue upon stimulation. As with any discovery there were the usual scoffers, and he became known as "the frog's dancing master."

With the invention of the electromagnet in 1820, many laboratory experiments verified Galvani's findings. Then in 1872, Gabriel Lippmann introduced his capillary electrometer. Two wires from an exposed animal heart conducted the electrical difference between the two contact points.

The mercury in the capillary tube moved because of the change of surface tension at the junction of the mercury and dilute sulfuric acid.

Marey (perhaps you recall his sphygmograph) modified this four years later to make permanent photographic recordings of the animal heart's electrical efforts.

Augustus Waller of London was the first to record the human heart. Since opening the chest for a direct recording was out of the question, he devised a pair of electrodes of zinc-covered chamois leather moistened in brine to reduce skin resistance. These he strapped to the front and back of the chest, and the electrical potential difference was recorded for history on moving photographic paper in 1887.

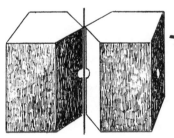

LIPPMANN'S CAPILLARY ELECTROMETER WITH MAREY'S PHOTOGRAPHIC RECORDER.

MERCURY

CHEST

SULFURIC ACID

CAPILLARY TUBE

CHEST

MOVING PHOTOGRAPHIC PLATE

Willen Einthoven, of Holland's Leiden University, found Lippmann's device sensitive, but unfortunately sluggish and erratic because of the inertia of the mercury. He had a better idea, and by 1901 had created the string galvanometer. Basically, the current from the heart ran down a fine silver-coated glass thread which was suspended between the two poles of an electromagnet. The shadow of the fluctuating string was projected onto a moving glass photographic plate for a permanent record.

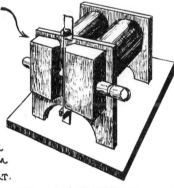

POLE PIECES OF EINTHOVEN'S ELECTROMAGNETS WITH SILVER COATED QUARTZ STRING FROM HIS DRAWINGS (ARCH. INTERNAT. PHYSIOL. 1906)

EINTHOVEN'S ELECTROMAGNET

The string galvanometer electrocardiogram was as large as its influence on twentieth century medicine. The original unit weighed six hundred pounds, and needed two rooms and five men to operate! With various improvements through the years, Einthoven's invention remains the basic unit in today's electocardiographs. It has yielded much of our present knowledge, and perhaps a brief review of the heart's electrical qualities would be in order.

Each resting heart muscle cell has a positively charged surface and a negatively charged interior. On excitation, the cell membrane becomes permeable to the surface's positively charged sodium ion (Na^+) which then crosses to the interior of the cell. The surface is now negatively charged and depolarized. The electrocardiogram measures the potential differential between this depolarized wave that is sweeping down the pathways of the heart and the still-resting positively charged cells ahead.

Electrodes and their wires (leads) from the right arm, left arm, left leg and chest (precordial) carry the electrical differential to charge the string of the galvanometer.

These multiple leads give a variety of recordings as the negative charge spreads out to contract the muscle cells. After Einthoven pondered the hills and valleys of the tracings, he arbitrarily chose letters from the middle of the alphabet for labeling.

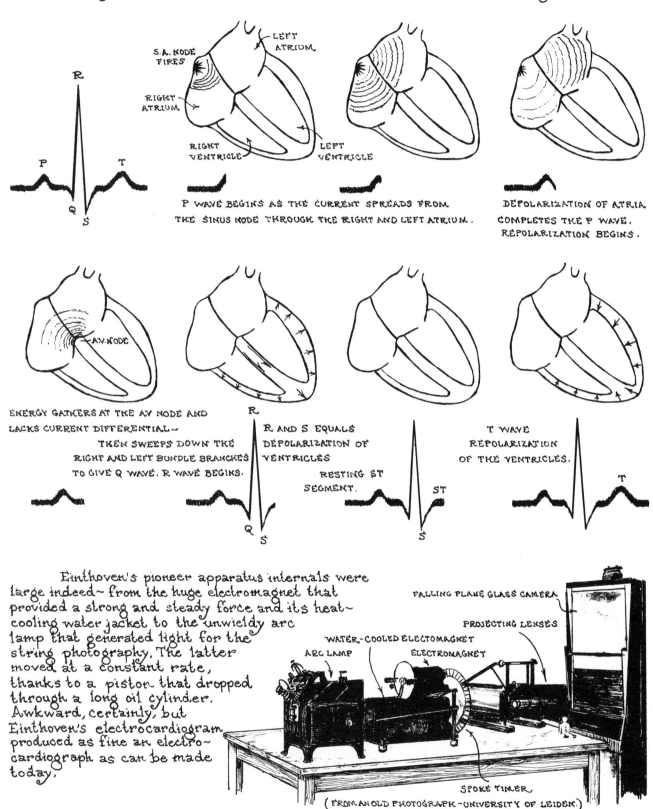

P WAVE BEGINS AS THE CURRENT SPREADS FROM THE SINUS NODE THROUGH THE RIGHT AND LEFT ATRIUM.

DEPOLARIZATION OF ATRIA COMPLETES THE P WAVE. REPOLARIZATION BEGINS.

ENERGY GATHERS AT THE AV NODE AND LACKS CURRENT DIFFERENTIAL~ THEN SWEEPS DOWN THE RIGHT AND LEFT BUNDLE BRANCHES TO GIVE Q WAVE. R WAVE BEGINS.

R AND S EQUALS DEPOLARIZATION OF VENTRICLES

RESTING ST SEGMENT.

T WAVE REPOLARIZATION OF THE VENTRICLES.

Einthoven's pioneer apparatus internals were large indeed~ from the huge electromagnet that provided a strong and steady force and its heat~cooling water jacket to the unwieldy arc lamp that generated light for the string photography. The latter moved at a constant rate, thanks to a piston that dropped through a long oil cylinder. Awkward, certainly, but Einthoven's electrocardiogram produced as fine an electro~cardiograph as can be made today.

FALLING PLANE GLASS CAMERA

PROJECTING LENSES

WATER-COOLED ELECTROMAGNET

ELECTROMAGNET

ARC LAMP

SPOKE TIMER

(FROM AN OLD PHOTOGRAPH~UNIVERSITY OF LEIDEN.)

EDELMANN AND SONS OF MUNICH AND THE CAMBRIDGE SCIENTIFIC INSTRUMENT COMPANY OF LONDON MODIFIED EINTHOVEN'S ORIGINAL ECG TO MAKE A MORE MANAGEABLE ECG. SIR THOMAS LEWIS USED THE 1908 CAMBRIDGE FOR HIS STUDIES OF ARRYTHMIAS.

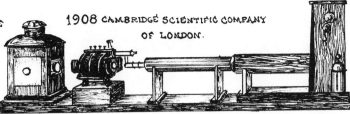

1908 CAMBRIDGE SCIENTIFIC COMPANY OF LONDON.

THE 100 PAPERS AND 3 BOOKS BY LEWIS SHOWED THE DIAGNOSTIC POSSIBILITIES OF THE ECG. THE 1909 EDELMANN MACHINE WAS THE FIRST TO BE BROUGHT TO AMERICA. IT WAS LESS ACCURATE THAN THE 1908 CAMBRIDGE BECAUSE OF THE TENDENCY OF THE "U" SHAPED GALVANOMETER POLES MOVING TOGETHER AND THROWING THE STRING OUT OF FOCUS.

1909 EDELMANN AND SONS OF MUNICH. DISPLAYED AT TULANE MEDICAL SCHOOL, NEW ORLEANS.

PROFESSOR HORATIO B. WILLIAMS VISITED EINTHOVEN, THEN RETURNED TO THE UNITED STATES TO DESIGN AN ECG. IN 1914, THE INSTRUMENT WAS BUILT BY CHARLES F. HINDLE ~ A MECHANIC AT THE OLD COLLEGE OF PHYSICIANS & SURGEONS OF N.Y.C. SOON AFTER THIS FIRST MACHINE TO BE BUILT IN THE U.S.A., HE FORMED THE HINDLE INSTRUMENT COMPANY TO PRODUCE 3 MODELS BETWEEN 1914 TO 1921.

CASE SLIDES OVER MOTOR.

1918 HINDLE INSTRUMENT COMPANY OF NEW YORK. ~ MODEL #2 ~ DISPLAYED AT MUTTER MUSEUM, COLLEGE OF PHYSICANS OF PHILADELPHIA.

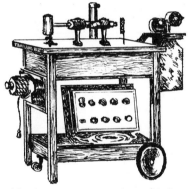

1921 HINDLE NO. 3 N.Y.C. IN 1922 THE HINDLE COMPANY OF NEW YORK BECAME THE CAMBRIDGE INSTRUMENT COMPANY OF AMERICA.

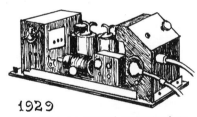

1929 CAMBRIDGE SCIENTIFIC INSTRUMENT COMPANY OF LONDON. 80 POUNDS AND MOVABLE.

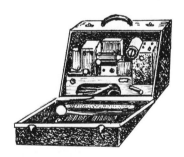

1928 CAMBRIDGE (LONDON). 30 POUNDS AND THE FIRST PORTABLE ELECTROCARDIOGRAM.

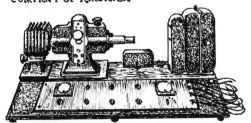

c.1930 BECK-LEE OFFICE MODEL WITH ONE OF THE FIRST PERMANENT STRING GALVANOMETERS

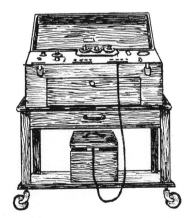

1930's VICTOR ECG BY GENERAL ELECTRIC WITH AMPLIFYING UNIT. U.S.A.

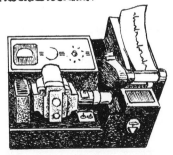

POST WORLD WAR II BECK-LEE CORPORATION, CHICAGO. INTRODUCED BUILT-IN DEVELOPING TANKS TO DEVELOP AN ELECTRO-CARDIOGRAM IN 4 SECONDS.

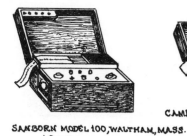

SANBORN MODEL 100, WALTHAM, MASS.

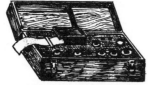

CAMBRIDGE "VERSA-SCRIBE," N.Y.C.

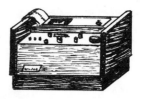

BECK-LEE "CARDIOMITE," CHICAGO.

c.1960 DIRECT-WRITING ELECTROCARDIOGRAPHS, PORTABLE (ALL THE ABOVE).

ELECTRODES

A gentleman was pictured in his pajamas and nightcap with a hand and a foot in buckets of water ~ or so it seemed ~ in one of the early photographs from Einthoven's 1906 article on electrodes and leads. Actually, the inventor of the string galvanometer was illustrating lead III electrodes for his electrocardiograph. The glass cylinder electrodes ~ electrolytic baths ~ were designed to carry the minute electrical currents from the heart through the skin barrier and into the galvanometer leads for recording.

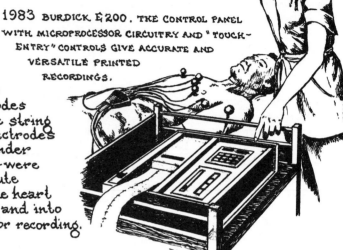

1983 BURDICK E200. THE CONTROL PANEL WITH MICROPROCESSOR CIRCUITRY AND "TOUCH-ENTRY" CONTROLS GIVE ACCURATE AND VERSATILE PRINTED RECORDINGS.

c 1906

→ TO A POLE OF GALVANOMETER.

← HAND IMMERSES IN INNER ZINC CYLINDER FILLED WITH SODIUM CHLORIDE.
← ZINC ELECTRODE.
← OUTER GLASS CYLINDER FILLED WITH ZINC SULFATE SOLUTION.

(EINTHOVEN, W., ARCH. INTERNAT. PHYSIO. 4:132, 1906)

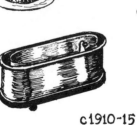

c 1910-15

FOOT AND HAND IMMERSION ELECTRODES.

By 1920, these wet-bath electrodes were has-beens with the introduction of strap~on electrodes by Cohn of the United States and Barron of England. As with the electrocardiographs, the electrodes had become more manageable and convenient.

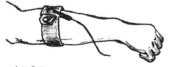

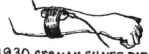

1930 GERMAN SILVER DIRECT CONTACT PLATE, CAMBRIDGE INSTRUMENT CO. OF NEW YORK.

c.1920 STRAP-ON ELECTRODES ~
COHN USED A RUBBER STRAP TO HOLD METAL FOIL IN CONTACT WITH THE SKIN. BARRON PREFERRED A FLEXIBLE COPPER MESH STRAP THAT WAS COVERED WITH FLANNEL AND SOAKED WITH AN ELECTROLYTIC SOLUTION.
(FROM "A HISTORY OF ELECTROCARDIOGRAPHY")

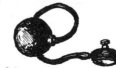

1932 BURGER'S SUCTION PRECORDIAL ELECTRODE.

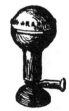

WELSH'S MODIFICATION OF BURGER'S ELECTRODE.

OPHTHALMOSCOPES

It was Jean Mery who first glimpsed the living retina—and under rather odd circumstances. In 1704 the Parisian anatomist held a cat under water! To his surprise, he could see the retinal details without difficulty. Since the technique lacked the niceties required when examining a patient's eye, no further observations were made until 1810. Until that date, it was generally believed that the red glare from an animal's eyes was generated from the nervous system. Not so, for Provost found no such glare in a darkened room. Reflection of light in the retina had to be the answer. This was verified by Cummings in 1846, who added the observation that it occured only when the observer's eye was in a direct line with the light

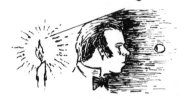

source and the patient's eye. More easily said than done, for if the light were between the examiner's and the patient's eye, the brightness would be dazzling. If placed in line with the patient's eye but behind the examiner's head, the light would be blocked.

For the while, physicians had to be content to inspect only the exterior eye. A large convex object lens was used to concentrate a bright spot of light over the eye's surface to check for uneveness, foreign bodies or opacities, corneal inflammation and abnormalities of the anterior chamber, iris or lens.

Any unusual finding was magnified by about four diameters with a compound folding lens. With the same hand, a finger elevated the patient's upper lid. The other hand held the object lens to give added brightness from the light source.

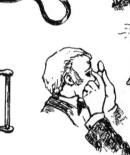

THE REFLECTING OPHTHALMOSCOPES

HELMHOLTZ—The mysteries deep within the eye continued to confound the medical profession. Meanwhile, a young German physician began his appointment to teach physiology and pathology at Königsberg in 1849. Hermann Helmholtz, in one of his lectures on the eye, demonstrated how light rays entered the pupil and then were reflected back as a red glow—and in the same pathways as those entering. If he could but devise an instrument that would place his own vision in line with those rays entering and leaving the patient's eye, its dark interior would yield its secrets.

One year later, at the age of twentynine, he wrote his father that "...it seems almost ludicrous that I and others should have been so slow to see it." Of his discovery, he went on to say "It is namely, a combination of glasses by means of which it is possible to illuminate the dark background of the eye, through the pupil, without employing any dazzling light, and to obtain a view of all the elements of the retina at once, more exactly than one can see the external parts of the eye without magnification..."

Helmholtz had sandwiched a concave lens, coverglasses and side pieces of cardboard. Light reflected off its slanted surface and into the patient's eye, returning through the clear glass to his own retina. His

1850 HELMHOLTZ

his monograph of 1851 described his exploration of the eye in detail along with diagrams of the actual instrument. Various concave lenses could be inserted to bring the retina into better focus, be it a near, normal or farsighted individual.

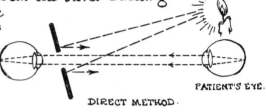

THE CONCAVE LENS MAGNIFIED THE RETINAL RAYS.

3 COVER GLASSES REFLECTED LIGHT.

PATIENT'S EYE.

Just two months after Helmholtz's, Epkins of Amsterdam made a surprisingly simple improvement. Using a flat mirror as a light reflector instead of Helmholtz's glass plates, he scraped off a small oval from the silver backing to act as a peephole. These reflecting ophthalmoscopes yielded a virtual erect image of the retina ~ the direct method ~ that could be enlarged to about fourteen times if a convex lens were inserted and the observer's eye was close to that of the patient.

1851 EPKINS

DIRECT METHOD.

PATIENT'S EYE.

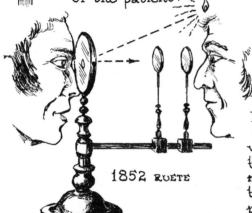

1852 RUETE

INDIRECT METHOD.

PATIENT'S EYE

In 1852 Ruéte of Göttingen used a concave mirror ~ with a hole drilled through its center ~ to concentrate the light rays. Further, he championed the indirect method for examining the eye by placing one or two convex lenses between the mirror and the patient. The result was an inverted picture of the retina. Although it gave a smaller image, the method gave an overall birdseye view and was generally used for a general idea of the fundus before using the direct method. Ophthalmoscopic sets of this period included convex lenses for this purpose.

Obviously, a good deal of juggling was necessary if one were to use the various concave lenses for the indirect visualization and the assorted concave lenses necessary for enlarged and clear images with the direct method. A mechanic in Helmholtz's home town, Mr. E. Rekoss, placed a series of small concave lenses into two revolving discs. When attached to the Helmholtz base (with the blessings of the doctor) the proper lens could be quickly found that would correct the physician's view for crystal ~ clear viewing. No need for spectacles here.

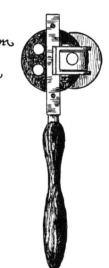

In 1853, Coccius concentrated light with a swinging arm biconvex condensing lens onto a flat square mirror. A later model, shown here, replaced the mirror with a thin metal flat mirror. Behind it was attached a clip to hold either concave or convex lenses to clarify the retinal image. Later still, a sliding bar of lenses was substituted for the clip. All in all, it lacked the convenience of the Rekoss disc.

1852 HELMHOLTZ WITH REKOSS DISC.

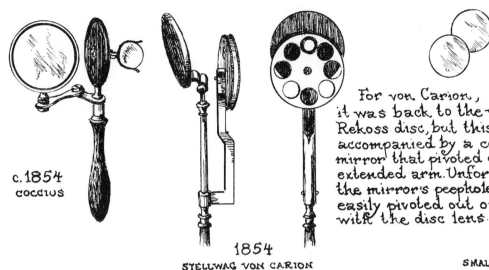

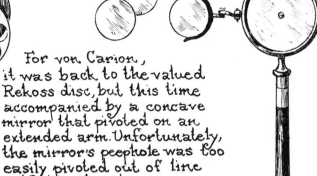

c. 1854
COCCIUS

For von Carion, it was back to the valued Rekoss disc, but this time accompanied by a concave mirror that pivoted on an extended arm. Unfortunately, the mirror's peephole was too easily pivoted out of line with the disc lens.

1854
STELLWAG VON CARION

1855
LIEBREICH'S
SMALL OPHTHALMOSCOPE.

Liebreich's small ophthalmoscope combined Reute's concave perforated mirror with Coccius' lens clips. Cased with the instrument were several concave and convex lenses to correct the refractive variations of the examiner's eye. Also included was a larger biconcave lens for indirect ophthamology. Unlike Coccius' model, this lens was held by the physician and not part of the ophthalmoscope.

The simplicity of Liebreich's model made it the favorite in Europe for over fifty years. It was so in America until Loring revived the Rekoss disc.

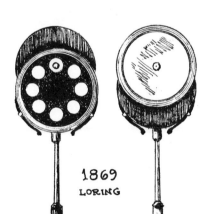

DIRECT OPHTHALMOSCOPY

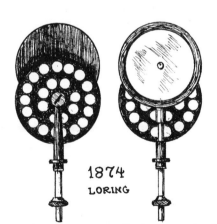

INDIRECT OPHTHALMOSCOPY

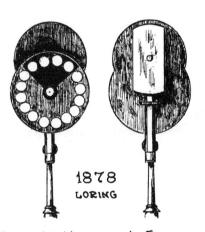

1869
LORING

1874
LORING

1878
LORING

In 1869, Dr. Edward G. Loring of New York City brought the search for a better ophthalmoscope to America. His first effort was a return to the disc of lenses idea, but unlike Rokoss', three detachable discs were used. One held a series of eight convex lenses, another eight concave, and the third eight were high powered assortments of both. The wide choice of lenses was a plus, but fumbling with all those discs was not.

The 1874 model boasted of twenty-three lenses in a single revolving disc. This was a workable arrangement and became immediately popular in the states. And so it would have remained had not Dr. O.F. Wadsworth of Boston observed three years later that the Loring mirror was fixed parallel to the disc of lenses. To reflect light, the mirror must be tilted toward the source ~ and the lens with it. Therefore, the image returning from the examined retina was necessarily distorted.

Loring immediately redesigned his ophthalmoscope, and in 1878 incorporated a long mirror that pivoted side-to-side. Further, he decreased the number of discs to sixteen of the most used. A secondary set of four lenses in a movable quadrant added to its versatility when superimposed on the Rekoss disc. Other instrument makers followed this innovation and the Loring was the preferred ophthalmoscope well into the early twentieth century.

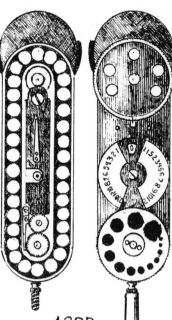

SWINGING MIRROR

1883
COUPER'S
CHAIN OF LENSES.

1883
MORTON'S
CHAIN OF LENSES

In 1883, John Couper of London produced an ingenious ophthalmoscope containing a continuous circuit of seventy-two lenses, each rolling freely on its neighbors. This circle of lenses moved around by means of a toothed wheel within the handle. Each lens was numbered and could be read through the sight-hole. A swinging mirror was located opposite the sight-hole.

A. S. Morton, also of London, liked Couper's ideas ~ so much, in fact, that he introduced his own modified version that very year. His series of twenty-nine lenses, rimmed with metal rings, moved when the lower disc and its interior toothed wheel were rotated with the finger. This disc also had black painted circles for comparison with the patient's pupils. The middle disc indicated the strength of the lens appearing at the sight-hole, while the upper disc of supplimentary lenses gave added lens power when needed.

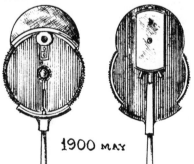

1900 MAY

America shrugged off the innovative Chain of lenses concept and continued with the Loring. In 1900, Charles H. May of New York City modified this favorite with fifteen concave and fifteen convex interchangeable lens discs.

ELECTRIC OPHTHALMOSCOPES

By the mid 1870's, the reflecting ophthalmoscope had earned its place alongside those diagnostic giants, the microscope, percussion hammer and the stethoscope. In America, the Loring seemed to have reached the pinnacle of perfection. It was a tidy, easily carried instrument with a convenient wheel of convex and concave lenses at one's fingertip.

If the viewer and patient both had normal vision (emmetropic), no lens was needed and the retina became clear with the proper selection in the concave lens series. A far-sighted eye (hypermetropic), would require the proper strength of the convex lens group. And if the physician were other than emmetropic, he need only wheel his lenses until the retina was no longer blurred.

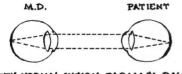

BOTH NORMAL VISION. PARALLEL RAYS NEED NO CONVERGENCE OR DIVERGENCE.

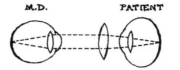

A NEARSIGHTED PATIENT REQUIRED A CONVEX LENS TO FOCUS ON CLOSER RETINA.

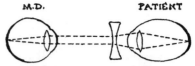

A FARSIGHTED PATIENT REQUIRED A CONCAVE LENS TO FOCUS ON DISTANT RETINA.

The movable reflecting mirror could throw a bright light into the eye's orbit if given a reasonable source. How could one improve on such an instrument? The inventive genius of Edison had the answer—the electric light bulb. It had become a reality in 1879 and there were several attempts to adapt the ophthalmoscope to the invention. Only when a bulb could be produced that was powerful yet small enough—and lighted with its own electrical power—would the Loring meet its master.

The credit for introducing the first electric ophthalmoscope belongs to Dr. W.S. Dennett of New York City. At the early date of 1885, he demonstrated the instrument before the American Ophthalmological Society. Looking much like a pen with an end flap, the small bulb in the handle was wired to a hefty battery. A convex lens concentrated light onto the angled mirror, then reflected into the patient's eye. Unfortunately, the bulb's carbon filament quickly expired, and the physician was likely to follow suit if he attempted to make the battery portable.

One year later, ophthamologist Thomas Reid of Glasgow introduced an electric ophthalmoscope that contained the bulb in a rather novel handle. By sliding the handle in and out of the prism tube, the light could be adjusted for the most concentrated retinal light reflection.

INTERCHANGEABLE REFLECTING MIRRORS.

1886 JULER'S ELECTRIC OPHTHALMOSCOPE.

TO BATTERY.   TO BATTERY.

1885 DENNETT.

Also in 1886, ophthamologist Henry Juler of London included a single disc of nine convex and fifteen concave lenses in his electrified version. The bulb was secured on the outside rather than the inside of the handle. Although the bulb had the early burn-out problems, the battery was of the smaller type used in telegraphy and more easily managed. There was added insurance if either failed—two concave mirrors that could be substituted for the electrical head. The larger was for indirect viewing, while the smaller was used for direct visualization.

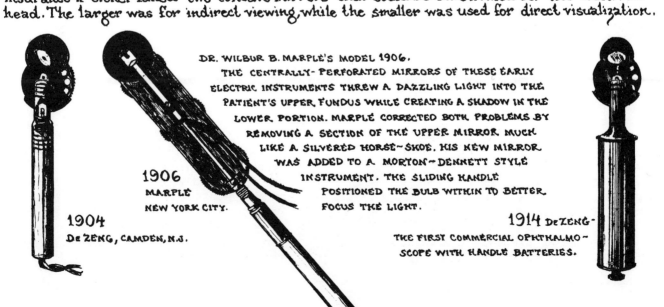

DR. WILBUR B. MARPLE'S MODEL 1906.
THE CENTRALLY-PERFORATED MIRRORS OF THESE EARLY ELECTRIC INSTRUMENTS THREW A DAZZLING LIGHT INTO THE PATIENT'S UPPER FUNDUS WHILE CREATING A SHADOW IN THE LOWER PORTION. MARPLE CORRECTED BOTH PROBLEMS BY REMOVING A SECTION OF THE UPPER MIRROR MUCH LIKE A SILVERED HORSE-SHOE. HIS NEW MIRROR WAS ADDED TO A MORTON-DENNETT STYLE INSTRUMENT. THE SLIDING HANDLE POSITIONED THE BULB WITHIN TO BETTER FOCUS THE LIGHT.

1906 MARPLE NEW YORK CITY.

1904 De ZENG, CAMDEN, N.J.

1914 DeZENG
THE FIRST COMMERCIAL OPHTHALMO- SCOPE WITH HANDLE BATTERIES.

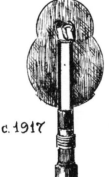

DR. CHARLES H. MAY. MAY'S 1900 REFLECTING OPHTHALMOSCOPE MAY HAVE BEEN OUT-DATED BY THE FLURRY OF ELECTRIC INSTRUMENTS ~ BUT IT WAS NOT FORGOTTEN, AT LEAST BY THE INVENTOR. IN 1914, HE UPDATED THE PIECE WITH BATTERIES AND A TINY BULB WITHIN THE HANDLE. HERE WAS A NEW CONCEPT IN LIGHT TRANSMISSION. A CONVEX LENS JUST ABOVE THE BULB CONCEN~ TRATED THE RAYS INTO A SOLID GLASS ROD. ITS UPPER PORTION WAS BEVELED AND SILVERED TO REFLECT INTO THE PATIENT'S EYE. THIS REFLECTING SURFACE COVERED ONLY THE LOWER HALF OF THE SIGHT-HOLE, THE UPPER PORTION OF THE HOLE REMAINING FREE TO RECEIVE THE REFLECTED LIGHT FROM THE RETINA. THE DISTANCE BETWEEN THE BULB AND THE BEVELED GLASS ROD COULD BE VARIED FOR LIGHT CONVER~ GENCE WITH A FINGER-CONTROLLED RHEOSTAT. MAY'S SUPERIOR LIGHTING SYSTEM REMAINS POPULAR TODAY.

1914
MAY ~ N.Y.C.

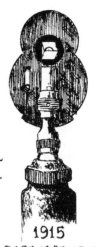

1915
DE ZENG "SIMPLEX"
REPLACED ITS EARLIER ROUND MIRROR WITH A SQUARE ONE. THE LENS DIAL CONTAINED 18 CONVEX AND CONCAVE LENSES. HANDLE BATTERIES.

1915
WELCH AND ALLYN
THE PROJECTING LIGHT BULB NEEDED NO REFLECTING SYSTEM, BUT THE GLARE MADE VISUALIZATION DIFFICULT. HANDLE BATTERIES.

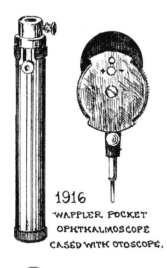

1916
WAPPLER POCKET OPHTHALMOSCOPE CASED WITH OTOSCOPE.

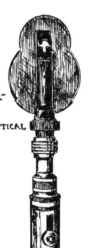

c.1917
DE ZENG ~ WITH MARPLE'S NOTCHED METAL MIRROR. POPULAR THROUGH THE 1930's.

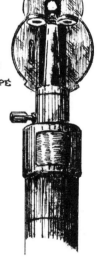

c.1920
"WELLSWORTH-DE ZENG" AMERICAN OPTICAL

COMBINED MARPLE'S MIRROR WITH THE DE ZENG HEAD. A SLIDING COLLAR MOVED THE LIGHT BULB TO GIVE A WIDE OR NARROW BEAM.

c.1925
GIANTSCOPE

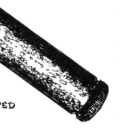

1928
FRIEDENWALD.

JONAS S. FRIEDENWALD OF THE JOHNS HOPKINS UNIVERSITY DEPARTMENT OF PATHOLOGY SCIENTIFICALLY DESIGNED A FOOT LONG INSTRUMENT (A REAL "GIANTSCOPE"!) THAT CONTAINED MANY REFINEMENTS IN APERTURES, FILTERS AND MAGNIFICATIONS. IT PROVED TO BE TOO LARGE AND COMPLICATED AN OPHTHALMOSCOPE FOR GENERAL USE.

GIANTSCOPE, AMERICAN OPTICAL COMPANY. BASICALLY OF THE DE ZENG DESIGN, IT WAS MORE "GIANT" FOR ITS HIGH-INTENSITY LIGHT THAN ITS SIZE. SUCH BRIGHTNESS WAS FELT A REAL PLUS FOR VISUALIZING PATHOLOGY THROUGH THE POLAROID, RED-FREE AND YELLOW MONOCHROMATIC FILTERS. YET IT WAS A BIT TOO STRONG FOR THE ROUTINE EXAMINATION, AND THE WIRES TO THE TRANSFORMER HAD A FRUS-TRATING WAY OF WEARING OUT.

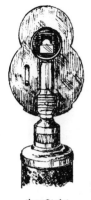

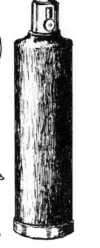

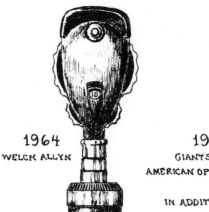

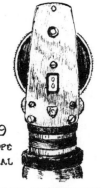

1920's

SIMPLEX
AMERICAN OPTICAL

LOOK-ALIKES OF THE 20's, CASED WITH AN OTOSCOPE. WELCH ALLYN ALSO JOINED THE LORING~MAY TREND IN 1932.

BAUSCH & LOMB

1964
WELCH ALLYN

THIS NEW DESIGN FEATURED A REFLECTING METAL MIRROR AND MULTIPLE APERTURES, RED-FREE LIGHT AND GRID. PRACTICAL.

1969
GIANTSCOPE
AMERICAN OPTICAL

IN ADDITION TO THE BRILLIANT LIGHT AND THE FILTERS, APERTURES AND LENS DISCS OF THE EARLIER VERSION, A COBALT BLUE FILTER FOR FLOURSCEIN STUDY AND A RHEOSTAT HANDLE CONTROL GAVE MORE VERSATILITY.

In 1891, Hermann von Helmholz, the originator of the ophthalmoscope, recalled in an address that "After previous investigation of the problem in all directions... happy ideas come unexpectedly without effort, like an inspiration." One such was the rechargeable battery handle of the early 1960's, and the more recent 3.5 volt halogen bulb. The natural white light, high intensity and a double longevity has made the old incandescent bulb obsolete.

TONOMETERS

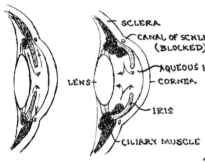

SCLERA
CANAL OF SCHLEMM (BLOCKED)
AQUEOUS HUMOR
LENS
CORNEA
IRIS
CILIARY MUSCLE

NORMAL EYE   GLAUCOMA

Glaucoma is an increase of intraocular tension. The anterior eye cavity is bathed and nourished by fluid (aqueous humor) from the ciliary body. The fluid escapes through a small opening (canal of Schlemm) at the angle formed by the iris and cornea. If this angle were blocked by such as adhesions or swelling, the fluid builds up a tension that may well destroy the vision.

In the 1920's, much of the credit for investigating aqueous humor secretions and circulation belonged to Jonas Friedenwald of Baltimore. His ophthalmoscope was previously noted.

The old timers resorted to "tactus eruditus"~a fancy term for estimating the intraocular tension by finger pressure over the closed lid. To give a more impartial and accurate reading, Rubino modified the Bloch-Verdin sphygmometer for this purpose. Because an increased pressure in the retinal arteries was believed to be an important contributor to intra-ocular tension, Rubino applied enough pressure to interrupt the retinal circulation. This point was supposedly reached when the eye temporarily lost its sight (!) and the recorded pressure was believed to be the same as that within the eye.

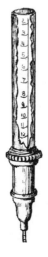

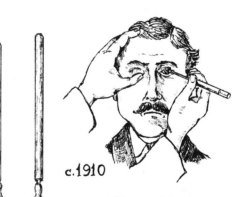

c.1910

RUBINO'S MODIFIED BLOCH-VERDIN SPHYGMOMANOMETER WITH SEVERAL FOOTED RODS.

In the early 1900's, the Stephenson tonometer made its brief debut. Pressure was exerted over the closed upper lid, and in turn was transmitted to an inner rod and its attached spring. The pressure was read from the scale on the barrel. A handle positioned the instrument over the patient's face. It had its problems, for it was difficult to know how much tension was intra-ocular and how much from the eyelid.

Schiotz experimented with his version of a tonometer between 1905 to 1911. The intra-ocular pressure was measured by the depth of depression made on the anesthetized cornea made by its weighted shaft. The greater the tension in the anterior chamber of the eye, the firmer the cornea and the higher the reading. Normal pressure was 20 mm. Hg, but any reading above 26 mm. Hg. spelled trouble. The Schiotz tonometer became an immediate favorite~ and remains so today.

(ALL BELOW FROM MUELLER & CO., 1929)

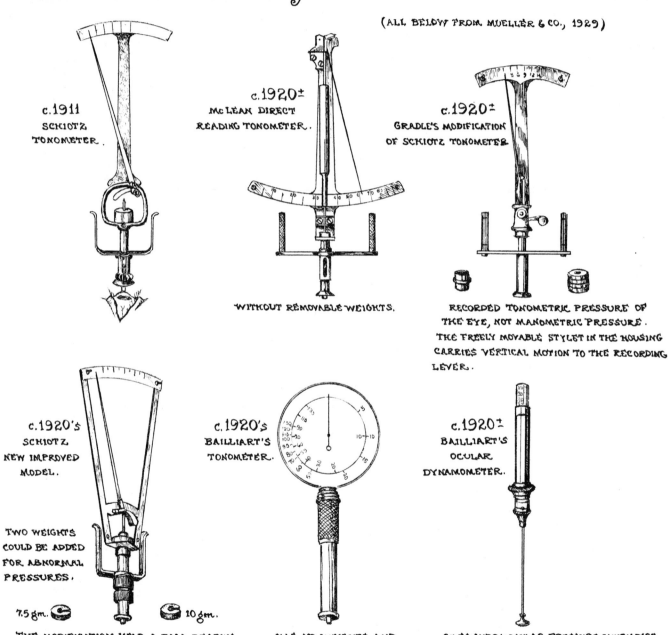

c.1911
SCHIOTZ
TONOMETER.

c.1920±
McLEAN DIRECT
READING TONOMETER.

WITHOUT REMOVABLE WEIGHTS.

c.1920±
GRADLE'S MODIFICATION
OF SCHIOTZ TONOMETER.

RECORDED TONOMETRIC PRESSURE OF
THE EYE, NOT MANOMETRIC PRESSURE.
THE FREELY MOVABLE STYLET IN THE HOUSING
CARRIES VERTICAL MOTION TO THE RECORDING
LEVER.

c.1920's
SCHIOTZ
NEW IMPROVED
MODEL.

TWO WEIGHTS
COULD BE ADDED
FOR ABNORMAL
PRESSURES.

7.5 gm.   10 gm.

THE MODIFICATION HELD A BALL BEARING
INSTEAD OF A COMMON SHAFT BEARING. IN
ADDITION, A 5.5 GRAM WEIGHT WAS FIXED TO
THE SHAFT FOR NORMAL EYE MEASUREMENT.

c.1920's
BAILLIART'S
TONOMETER.

HAS NO WEIGHTS AND
WORKS EQUALLY WELL IN
VERTICAL OR HOROZONTAL
POSITION.

c.1920±
BAILLIART'S
OCULAR
DYNAMOMETER.

GIVES INTRA-OCULAR PRESSURE. WHEN DISC
PRESSURE CAUSES RETINAL PULSE TO APPEAR,
DIASTOLIC PRESSURE IS READ, PRESSING UNTIL
PULSE DISAPPEARS GIVES SYSTOLIC PRESSURE.

THE OTOSCOPE

Until the early 1800's, one's ears were regarded as little more than bilateral scoops that funneled sound down a dark passageway to the ear drum. Gaspard Itard of Provence first stirred interest in the subject with his treatise on diseases of the ear in 1821. Adam Politzer followed up by popularizing the otoscope with his atlas – its high-point being the appearance of the membrana tympani by illumination.

The early otoscope was simplicity itself. The cone-shaped tube, according to Samuel Cooper's 1832 Dictionary of Practical Surgery, was placed in the ear canal while the left hand pulled outwards and upwards so as to elongate the cartelagenous portion of the canal. The direct rays of the sun were necessary unless one had the good fortune to focus a decent lantern in a darkened room.

In the America of 1883, according to Pomeroy, the Toynbee speculum was easily inserted and positioned for viewing. Its funnel shape, however, made surgery difficult. Gruber's otoscope bulged at its outer portion and was more roomy for this purpose. To some extent, the early Wilde speculum combined both these advantages.

As for the bivalve specula, they were little used except for a "few instances when operating." Kramer's, or Speer's "are as good as any" as well as Miliken's Self-Retaining Speculum. The more complicated reflecting instruments such as Hinton's and Brunston's were considered useful but rather needless crutches.

The following instruments, illustrated in various medical catalogues and textbooks, give some indication of their popularity in America.

SIMPLE SPECULA ~ usually came in sets of three.

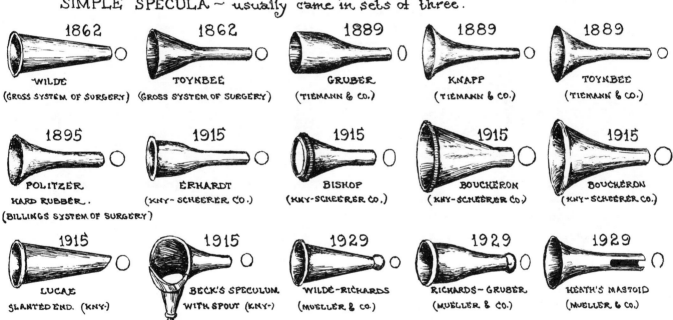

1862 WILDE (GROSS SYSTEM OF SURGERY)
1862 TOYNBEE (GROSS SYSTEM OF SURGERY)
1889 GRUBER (TIEMANN & CO.)
1889 KNAPP (TIEMANN & CO.)
1889 TOYNBEE (TIEMANN & CO.)

1895 POLITZER HARD RUBBER. (BILLINGS SYSTEM OF SURGERY)
1915 ERHARDT (KNY-SCHEERER CO.)
1915 BISHOP (KNY-SCHEERER CO.)
1915 BOUCHERON (KNY-SCHEERER CO.)
1915 BOUCHERON (KNY-SCHEERER CO.)

1915 LUCAE SLANTED END. (KNY.)
1915 BECK'S SPECULUM WITH SPOUT (KNY-)
1929 WILDE-RICHARDS (MUELLER & CO.)
1929 RICHARDS-GRUBER (MUELLER & CO.)
1929 HEATH'S MASTOID (MUELLER & CO.)

BIVALVE SPECULA ~ used in America since the early nineteenth century.

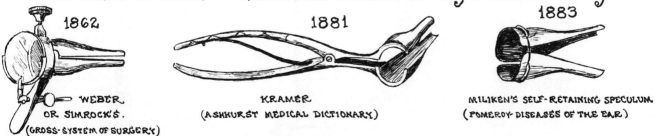

1862 WEBER OR SIMROCK'S. (GROSS SYSTEM OF SURGERY)
1881 KRAMER (ASHHURST MEDICAL DICTIONARY)
1883 MILIKEN'S SELF-RETAINING SPECULUM. (POMEROY-DISEASES OF THE EAR)

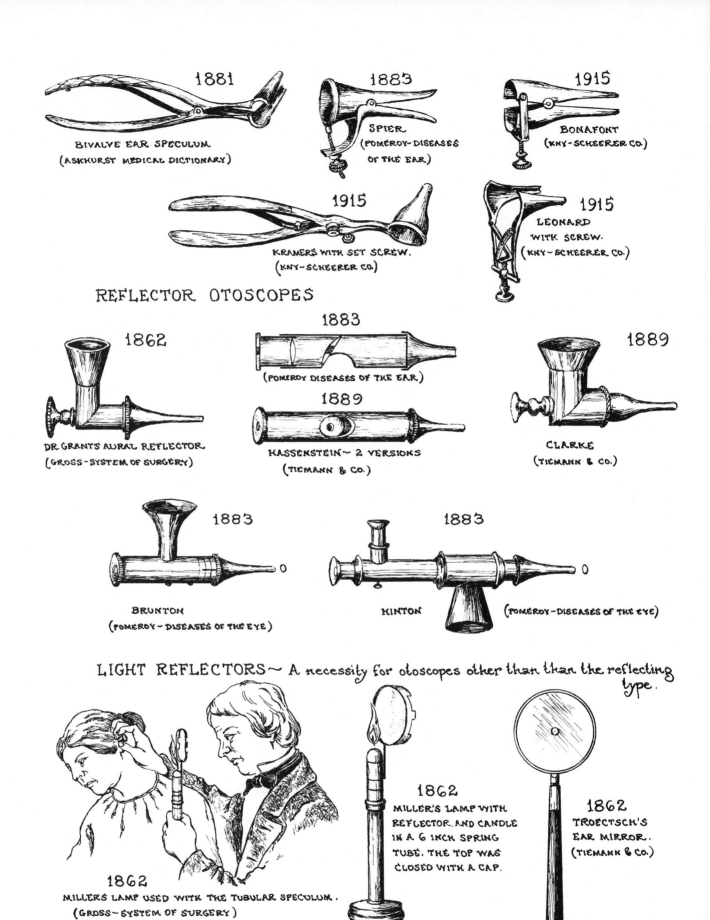

1881
BIVALVE EAR SPECULUM
(ASHHURST MEDICAL DICTIONARY)

1883
SPIER
(POMEROY-DISEASES
OF THE EAR)

1915
BONAFONT
(KNY-SCHEERER CO.)

1915
KRAMER'S WITH SET SCREW.
(KNY-SCHEERER CO.)

1915
LEONARD
WITH SCREW.
(KNY-SCHEERER CO.)

REFLECTOR OTOSCOPES

1862
DR. GRANT'S AURAL REFLECTOR.
(GROSS-SYSTEM OF SURGERY)

1883
(POMEROY DISEASES OF THE EAR)

1889
HASSENSTEIN~ 2 VERSIONS
(TIEMANN & CO.)

1889
CLARKE
(TIEMANN & CO.)

1883
BRUNTON
(POMEROY - DISEASES OF THE EYE)

1883
HINTON
(POMEROY-DISEASES OF THE EYE)

LIGHT REFLECTORS~ A necessity for otoscopes other than than the reflecting type.

1862
MILLERS LAMP USED WITH THE TUBULAR SPECULUM.
(GROSS-SYSTEM OF SURGERY)

1862
MILLER'S LAMP WITH
REFLECTOR. AND CANDLE
IN A 6 INCH SPRING
TUBE. THE TOP WAS
CLOSED WITH A CAP.

1862
TROECTSCH'S
EAR MIRROR.
(TIEMANN & CO.)

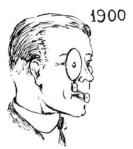

1900

HEAD MIRROR SUPPORTED
BY TEETH.
(APPLETON'S MEDICAL
LIBRARY, N.Y.)

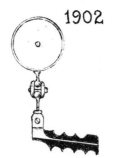

1902

REFLECTOR WITH MOUTH-
PLATE (AFTER LUCAE)
(BRUKL-ATLAS AND EPITOME
OF OTOLOGY)

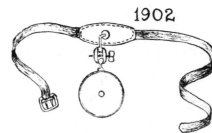

1902

HEAD MIRROR (AFTER HARLMAN)
(BRUKL-ATLAS AND EPITOME
OF OTOLOGY)

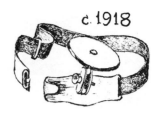

c.1918

GLEASON
WITH LEATHER STRAP.
(F. K. THOMAS CO.)

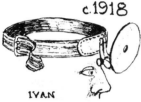

c.1918

IVAN
(F.H. THOMAS CO.)

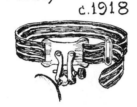

c.1918

BOSWORTH
(F. H. THOMAS CO.)

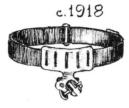

c.1918

SCHROETTER
(F. K. THOMAS CO.)

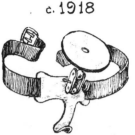

c.1918

HASLAM'S WITH NOSE REST.
(F. H. THOMAS CO.)

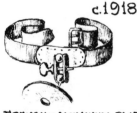

c.1918

FRENCH-ALUMINUM PLATE.
(F. H. THOMAS CO.)

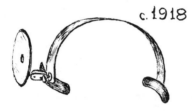

c.1918

WORRELL'S STEEL SPRING.
(F. K. THOMAS CO.)

The minor differences between these reflecting mirrors may seem less than exciting today, particularly since the small electrical head lamp had already elbowed its way into the turn-of-the century medical catalogues. Yet reflected light was considered superior for visualizing the deeper recesses of the ear.

This was emphasized by Brüll and Smith in their 1902 <u>Atlas and Epitome of Otology</u>. They then went on to describe the ideal concave mirror as being fifteen centimeters in diameter and having a focal distance of fifteen centimeters. It could be held in the hand, or between the teeth, or attached to the forehead with an elastic or leather band. Each had its own version of the ball-and-socket joint to permit free motion in any direction. In use, the light source was placed at the level of the ear, to the right and somewhat behind the patient's head. With the mirror against the examiner's forehead and nose, the rays reflected from its surface at a forty five degree angle.

ELECTRIC OTOSCOPES

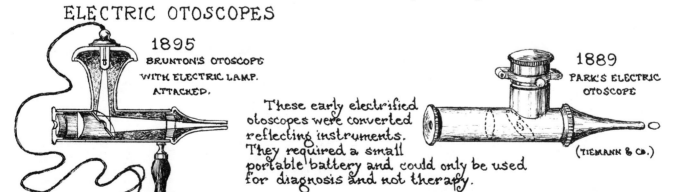

1895

BRUNTON'S OTOSCOPE
WITH ELECTRIC LAMP.
ATTACHED.

1889

PARK'S ELECTRIC
OTOSCOPE

(TIEMANN & CO.)

These early electrified otoscopes were converted reflecting instruments. They required a small portable battery and could only be used for diagnosis and not therapy.

(BILLING'S SYSTEM OF SURGERY)

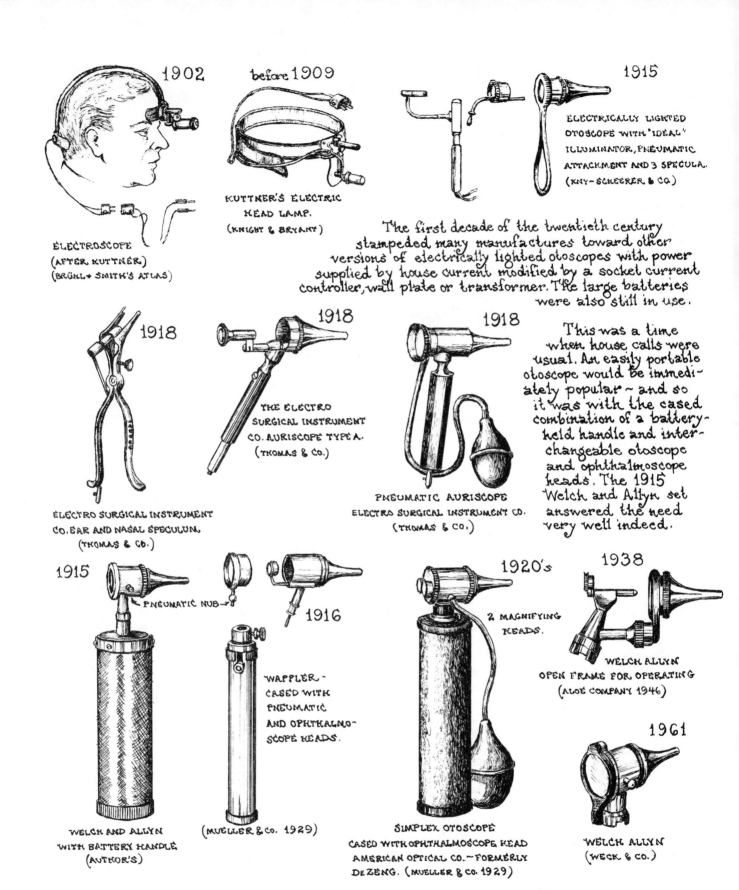

1902

ELECTROSCOPE
(AFTER KUTTNER)
(BRÜHL & SMITH'S ATLAS)

before 1909

KUTTNER'S ELECTRIC
HEAD LAMP.
(KNIGHT & BRYANT)

1915

ELECTRICALLY LIGHTED
OTOSCOPE WITH "IDEAL"
ILLUMINATOR, PNEUMATIC
ATTACHMENT AND 3 SPECULA.
(KNY-SCHEERER & CO.)

The first decade of the twentieth century stampeded many manufactures toward other versions of electrically lighted otoscopes with power supplied by house current modified by a socket current controller, wall plate or transformer. The large batteries were also still in use.

1918

ELECTRO SURGICAL INSTRUMENT
CO. EAR AND NASAL SPECULUM.
(THOMAS & CO.)

1918

THE ELECTRO
SURGICAL INSTRUMENT
CO. AURISCOPE TYPE A.
(THOMAS & CO.)

1918

PNEUMATIC AURISCOPE
ELECTRO SURGICAL INSTRUMENT CO.
(THOMAS & CO.)

This was a time when house calls were usual. An easily portable otoscope would be immediately popular ~ and so it was with the cased combination of a battery-held handle and interchangeable otoscope and ophthalmoscope heads. The 1915 Welch and Allyn set answered the need very well indeed.

1915

PNEUMATIC NUB →

WELCH AND ALLYN
WITH BATTERY HANDLE
(AUTHOR'S)

1916

WAPPLER -
CASED WITH
PNEUMATIC
AND OPHTHALMO-
SCOPE HEADS.

(MUELLER & CO. 1929)

1920's

2 MAGNIFYING
HEADS.

SIMPLEX OTOSCOPE
CASED WITH OPHTHALMOSCOPE HEAD
AMERICAN OPTICAL CO. ~ FORMERLY
DE ZENG. (MUELLER & CO. 1929)

1938

WELCH ALLYN
OPEN FRAME FOR OPERATING
(ALOE COMPANY 1946)

1961

WELCH ALLYN
(WECK & CO.)

By 1960, rechargeable battery handles began replacing the old C and D batteries.

The 3.5 volt, halogen-illuminated otoscope bulb of the 1970's has made the incandescent bulb obsolete. Its white light has eliminated the yellowish unnatural color of the ear drum, has three times the light intensity and lasts twice as long as the incandescent bulb.

THE PNEUMATIC OTOSCOPE

Whatever the choice from this great selection of aural speculae, no ear examination was complete without testing the mobility of the ear drum. Direct visualization, at best, could only diagnose sixty percent of those with fluid in the middle ear ~ otherwise known as acute otitis media with effusion or acute suppurative otitis media. Pneumatoscopy was the answer.

(DRUIT 1867)

c. 1850's

Early on, the afflicted patient might be aware of inner ear fluid buildup from sudden noises caused by the "bursting of mucous bubbles." (DRUIT) To verify this, the physician of the mid 1800's placed a "Toynbee's otoscope" stethoscope" into his ear and that of the patient. The patient then held his nose and attempted to blow through it. If his doctor heard a squealing or gurgling sound, fluid was indeed present.

(DRUIT 1867)

TOYNBEE'S OTOSCOPE (DRUIT)
HARVEY'S FLEXIBLE STETHOSCOPE DIFFERED
BY HAVING A HOLLOW BELL THAT WAS PLACED
OVER AND NOT IN THE PATIENT'S EAR.

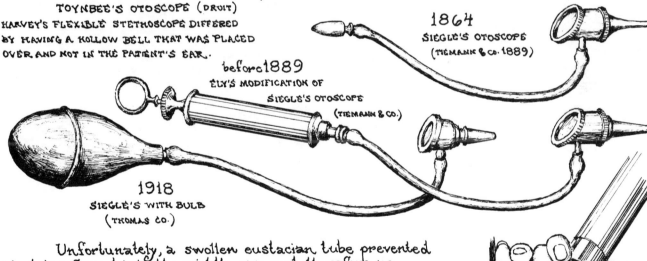

before 1889
ELY'S MODIFICATION OF
SIEGLE'S OTOSCOPE
(TIEMANN & CO.)

1864
SIEGLE'S OTOSCOPE
(TIEMANN & CO. 1889)

1918
SIEGLE'S WITH BULB
(THOMAS CO.)

Unfortunately, a swollen eustacian tube prevented air being forced into the middle ear, and therefore no characteristic bubbling sounds. Still, the Toynbee otoscope continued to be used in America into the 1940's.

In 1864, Siegle guaranteed a surer diagnosis with his pneumatic otoscope. By gently sucking in and then blowing out of the mouthpiece, the mobility of the drum could be observed directly. There would be no motion if fluid filled the middle ear. Siegle's discovery has stood the test of time, and the technique continues in use with our most up-to-date otoscopes.

EAR DRUM
EXTERNAL CANAL
MIDDLE EAR
EUSTACHIAN TUBE
NASOPHARYNX

1983

NASAL SPECULA

Nasal diagnostic instruments, like the aural, are either cone~shaped or bi-valved dilators. In general, those for rhinoscopy have less flare of the blades and are of a shorter length. Some are self~retaining, and inserted so that the blades press against the wall of the nose and septum, with the handle parallel to the floor. The ordinary nasal speculum, however, is inserted so that the blades are parallel to the floor of the nose. The index finger rests on the tip of the nose to steady the speculum as the blades are separated.

In the early 1800's, a simple bivalved dilator seemed adequate. By the 1870's, the instrument market erupted with a host of new versions that rarely escaped "improvements" in subsequent catalogues. This unbridled enthusiasm continued for upward to half a century. By the 1930's, most American physicians looked down their collective noses at the more outlandish types. As early as 1909, Knight stated flatly that "All fenestrated instruments, with uncontrolled springs, are to be condemned."

As with the otoscopes, the following specula date from their earliest catalogue availability or as recommended in textbooks of the period. Some found favor over extended periods, and their last catalogue appearance is noted. To better compare the changes in form and popularity, each example will be somewhat reduced in size and detail.

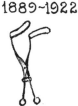
FROM 1800

BIVALVE
(ERICHSEN~SCIENCE + ART OF SURGERY 1869)

1865~1938

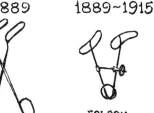
DUPLAY
(BOSWORTH~DISEASES OF NOSE AND THROAT 1881 TO MUELLER & CO. 1938)

1881~1946

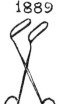
FRAENKEL
(BOSWORTH 1881 TO ALOE & CO. 1946)

1881~9

GOODWILLIE
(BOSWORTH 1881 TO TIEMANN & CO. 1889)

1881~1961

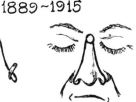
BOSWORTH
(BOSWORTH 1881 TO WECK & CO. 1961)

1881~1925

SIMROCK
(BOSWORTH 1881 TO WECK 1961)

1881~1915

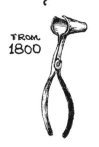
ELSBURG
(BOSWORTH 1881 TO KNY-SCHEERER CO 1915)

1889

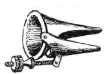
BONAFONT
(TIEMANN & CO. 1889)

1889

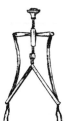
BIVALVE
(TIEMANN 1889)

1881~1915

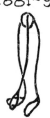
SHURLEY'S
WITH IVORY SLIDE
(BOSWORTH 1881 TO KNY 1915)

1889

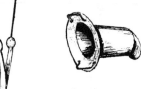
ROBERT AND COLLINS
(TIEMANN & CO. 1889)

1889

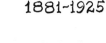
JARVIS OPERATING ~
RING SLIPS DOWN TO BECOME
SELF~RETAINING.
(TIEMANN & CO. 1889)

1889~1922

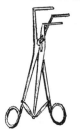
JARVIS
(TIEMANN & CO. 1889)

1889

SEXTON
(TIEMANN 1889)

1889~1915

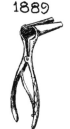
FOLSOM
(TIEMANN & CO. 1889 TO KNY-SCHEERER CO. 1915)

1889~1915

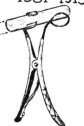
ANDREW H. SMITH
(TIEMANN & CO. 1889 TO KNY-SCHEERER CO. 1915)

1889~1915

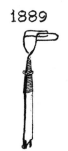
THUDICHUM
(TIEMANN & CO. 1889 TO KNY-SCHEERER 1915)

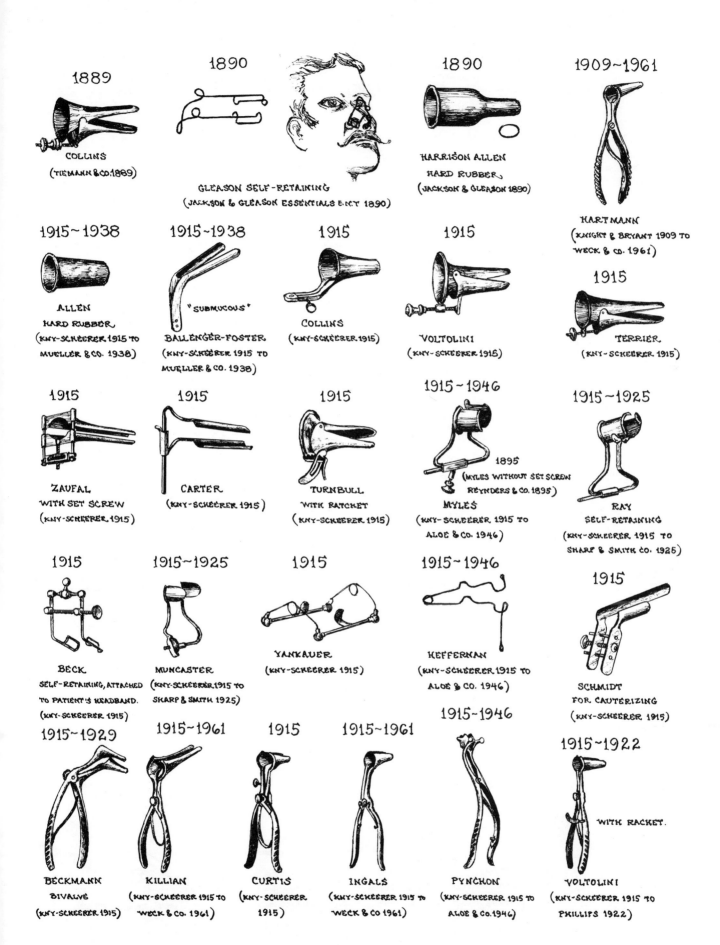

1889
COLLINS
(TIEMANN & CO. 1889)

1890
GLEASON SELF-RETAINING
(JACKSON & GLEASON ESSENTIALS E.N.T 1890)

1890
HARRISON ALLEN
HARD RUBBER
(JACKSON & GLEASON 1890)

1909~1961
HARTMANN
(KNIGHT & BRYANT 1909 TO
WECK & CO. 1961)

1915~1938
ALLEN
HARD RUBBER
(KNY-SCHEERER 1915 TO
MUELLER & CO. 1938)

1915~1938
"SUBMUCOUS"
BALLENGER-FOSTER
(KNY-SCHEERER 1915 TO
MUELLER & CO. 1938)

1915
COLLINS
(KNY-SCHEERER 1915)

1915
VOLTOLINI
(KNY-SCHEERER 1915)

1915
TERRIER
(KNY-SCHEERER 1915)

1915
ZAUFAL
WITH SET SCREW
(KNY-SCHEERER 1915)

1915
CARTER
(KNY-SCHEERER 1915)

1915
TURNBULL
WITH RATCHET
(KNY-SCHEERER 1915)

1915~1946
1895
(MYLES WITHOUT SET SCREW
REYNDERS & CO. 1895)
MYLES
(KNY-SCHEERER 1915 TO
ALOE & CO. 1946)

1915~1925
RAY
SELF-RETAINING
(KNY-SCHEERER 1915 TO
SHARP & SMITH CO. 1925)

1915
BECK
SELF-RETAINING, ATTACHED
TO PATIENT'S HEADBAND.
(KNY-SCHEERER 1915)

1915~1925
MUNCASTER
(KNY-SCHEERER 1915 TO
SHARP & SMITH 1925)

1915
YANKAUER
(KNY-SCHEERER 1915)

1915~1946
HEFFERNAN
(KNY-SCHEERER 1915 TO
ALOE & CO. 1946)

1915
SCHMIDT
FOR CAUTERIZING
(KNY-SCHEERER 1915)

1915~1929
BECKMANN
BIVALVE
(KNY-SCHEERER 1915)

1915~1961
KILLIAN
(KNY-SCHEERER 1915 TO
WECK & CO. 1961)

1915
CURTIS
(KNY-SCHEERER
1915)

1915~1961
INGALS
(KNY-SCHEERER 1915 TO
WECK & CO 1961)

1915~1946
PYNCHON
(KNY-SCHEERER 1915 TO
ALOE & CO. 1946)

1915~1922
WITH RACKET.
VOLTOLINI
(KNY-SCHEERER 1915 TO
PHILLIPS 1922)

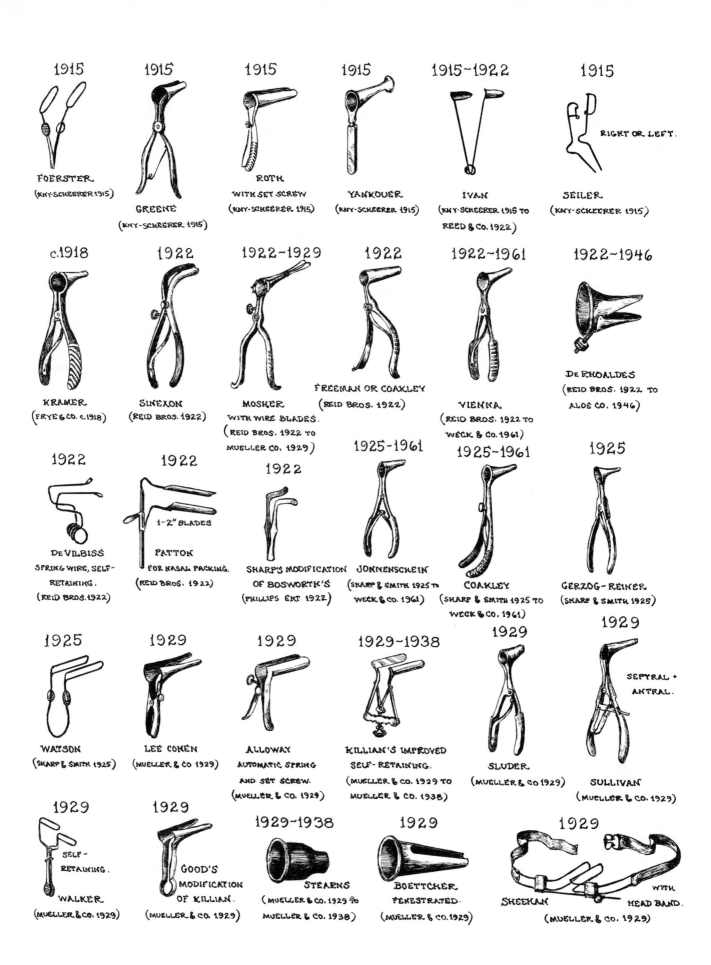

1915
FOERSTER
(KNY-SCHEERER 1915)

1915
GREENE
(KNY-SCHEERER 1915)

1915
ROTH
WITH SET SCREW
(KNY-SCHEERER, 1915)

1915
YANKOUER
(KNY-SCHEERER. 1915)

1915~1922
IVAN
(KNY-SCHEERER 1915 TO
REED & CO. 1922)

1915
RIGHT OR LEFT.
SEILER
(KNY-SCHEERER 1915)

c.1918
KRAMER
(FRYE & CO. c.1918)

1922
SINEXON
(REID BROS. 1922)

1922~1929
MOSHER
WITH WIRE BLADES.
(REID BROS. 1922 TO
MUELLER CO. 1929)

1922
FREEMAN OR COAKLEY
(REID BROS. 1922)

1922~1961
VIENNA
(REID BROS. 1922 TO
WECK & CO. 1961)

1922~1946
De RHOALDES
(REID BROS. 1922 TO
ALOE CO. 1946)

1922
DE VILBISS
SPRING WIRE, SELF-
RETAINING.
(REID BROS. 1922)

1922
1~2" BLADES
PATTON
FOR NASAL PACKING.
(REID BROS. 1922)

1922
SHARP'S MODIFICATION
OF BOSWORTH'S
(PHILLIPS ENT. 1922)

1925~1961
JONNENSCHEIN
(SHARP & SMITH 1925 TO
WECK & CO. 1961)

1925~1961
COAKLEY
(SHARP & SMITH 1925 TO
WECK & CO. 1961)

1925
GERZOG-REINER
(SHARP & SMITH 1925)

1925
WATSON
(SHARP & SMITH 1925)

1929
LEE COHEN
(MUELLER & CO 1929)

1929
ALLOWAY
AUTOMATIC SPRING
AND SET SCREW.
(MUELLER & CO. 1929)

1929~1938
KILLIAN'S IMPROVED
SELF-RETAINING.
(MUELLER & CO. 1929 TO
MUELLER & CO. 1938)

1929
SLUDER
(MUELLER & CO 1929)

1929
SEPTRAL +
ANTRAL.
SULLIVAN
(MUELLER & CO. 1929)

1929
SELF-
RETAINING.
WALKER
(MUELLER & CO. 1929)

1929
GOOD'S
MODIFICATION
OF KILLIAN.
(MUELLER & CO. 1929)

1929~1938
STEARNS
(MUELLER & CO. 1929 TO
MUELLER & CO. 1938)

1929
BOETTCHER
FENESTRATED.
(MUELLER & CO. 1929)

1929
SHEEHAN
WITH
HEAD BAND.
(MUELLER & CO. 1929)

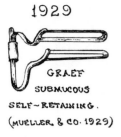

1929

GRAEF
SUBMUCOUS
SELF~RETAINING.
(MUELLER & CO. 1929)

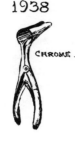

1938

CHROME.

LILLIE
(MUELLER & CO. 1939)

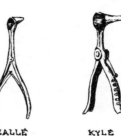

1961

HALLE
INFANT SPECULUM.
(WECK & CO 1961)

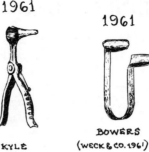

1961

KYLE
FOR CHILDREN.
(WECK & CO. 1961)

1961

BOWERS
(WECK & CO. 1961)

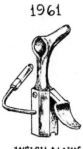

1961

WELCH ALLYN
ILLUMINATED NASAL
SPECULUM~ATTACHED TO HANDLE.
(WECK & CO. 1961)

MORE ON HEAD LAMPS

The reflecting head mirror and the electric head lamp competed for popularity during the first half of the twentieth century. Both were important for aural and nasal diagnosis, but lost ground with the introduction of the battery-in-handle otoscope~rhinoscope~ophthalmoscope combinations. Indeed, some medical catalogues listed the electric head lamp as a laryngoscope because of its increased use in that field.

The earlier electric head sets of the 1900~1920's (perhaps you recall the several under "otoscopes") remained basically unchanged. Klaar's model lost favor in the 1930's, while the Jansen and Kirstein versions held on through the 1950's. The "Ideal", looking much like a lighted elephant's trunk, was not all that the name implied. It was soon discarded.

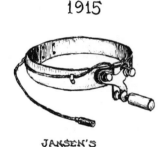

1915

JANSEN'S

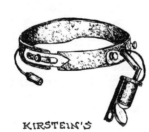

1915

KIRSTEIN'S

(ALL KNY-SCHEERER COMPANY 1915)

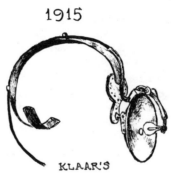

1915

KLAAR'S

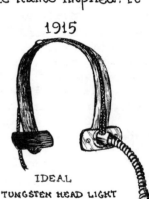

1915

IDEAL
TUNGSTEN HEAD LIGHT
WITH POCKET BATTERY.

The 1920's brought forth head lamps that looked more like floor lamps. Large and rather cumbersome, they gave a brilliant light that was appreciated by many physicians. By the 1950's, the trend was for less weighty lights that were smaller and more intense~and some with adjustable beams. The old and reliable reflecting head mirrors were without head lamp competition in the 1960's catalogues. Special-ized lighting systems for endoscopic examinations had taken over the field.

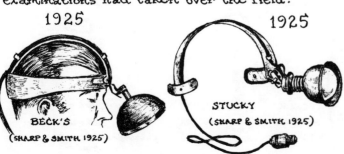

1925

BECK'S
(SHARP & SMITH 1925)

1925

STUCKY
(SHARP & SMITH 1925)

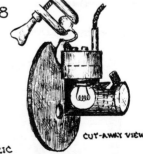

1938

CUT-AWAY VIEW

HASLINGER ELECTRIC
HEAD LAMP~CONCENTRATED LIGHT NEAR LINE OF VISION.
(MUELLER & CO. 1938)

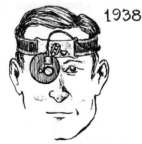

TONGUE DEPRESSORS

18TH CENTURY

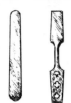

ENGLISH SILVER
(WELLCOME MUSEUM,
LONDON)

c.1850

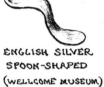

ENGLISH SILVER
SPOON-SHAPED
(WELLCOME MUSEUM)

AMERICAN IVORY AND
PRESSED HORN DEPRESSORS
(AUTHOR'S)

c.1840~50

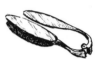

HINGED, PLATED
(AUTHOR'S)

1861

FOLDING DEPRESSOR
(GROSS~SYSTEM OF SURGERY
1862)

When the Pilgrims landed at Plymouth, the medical community back in mother England was just becoming aware of the diagnostic possibilities within the mouth. European and British physicians found a spatula useful for clearing the view obstructed by a troublesome tongue. By the eighteenth century, these were usually a heavy silver blade or a finely wrought silver instrument with intricately scrolled designs.

In America, apprentice-trained physicians made do with whatever was at hand. Likely they would have agreed with Dr. Samuel Gross a century later when he wrote in his 1862 System of Surgery, that reasonable tongue depressors were a "...book-folder, a wooden spatula, the handle of a spoon or a common grooved director."

The make-do-or-do-without throat stick was, however, receiving stiff competition even in Gross's day. The plain silver English spatula form was crafted from ivory or pressed horn in the early 1800's and silver plated steel was in use before the Civil War. Around 1840~1850, handles were added, while others were hinged space-savers.

Dr Francke H. Bosworth of Belleview Hospital was one of our outstanding early laryngologists. Although he stated in his 1881 Diseases of the Throat and Nose "There is no better instrument devised than the ordinary U.S. Army spatula" (although "rudely made"). His own tongue depressor design has remained popular through the decades.

Rust-resistant nickle plating surfaced many old styles in the 1880's when sterilization became widely practiced. Then came an explosion of new forms in the early 1900's. Minor changes were made in the Bosworth. The Andrews' and Wieder's designs of that period are among the few that are still appreciated and in use today.

TECHNIQUE ~ as described by Bosworth. The "beak" of the spatula should just cover the arch of the tongue, or the center will arch up and obstruct the inspection. Since the tongue is sensitive, pressure further back on the tongue may well produce retching or vomiting.

"The spatula should be held between the thumb and forefinger; the thumb, pressing against the angle while the second finger passes under the chin; in this manner a grasp is obtained of the lower jaw, and control of the movement of the head secured."

The tongue is pressed downward and forward with a slight rotary movement to see the pharynx.

1881

THE BOSWORTH IN ACTION.

c.1881

SEXTON'S SPATULA.
(BOSWORTH 1881)

c.1881

POCKET FOLDING
SPATULA
(BOSWORTH 1881)

c.1881

U.S. ARMY
(BOSWORTH 1881)

c.1881-15

TUERCK
(BOSWORTH
1881)

1881-15

SASS
(BOSWORTH 1881)

1890

FOLDING TONGUE
DEPRESSOR
(GLEASON-ESSENTIALS DISEASES ENT
1890)

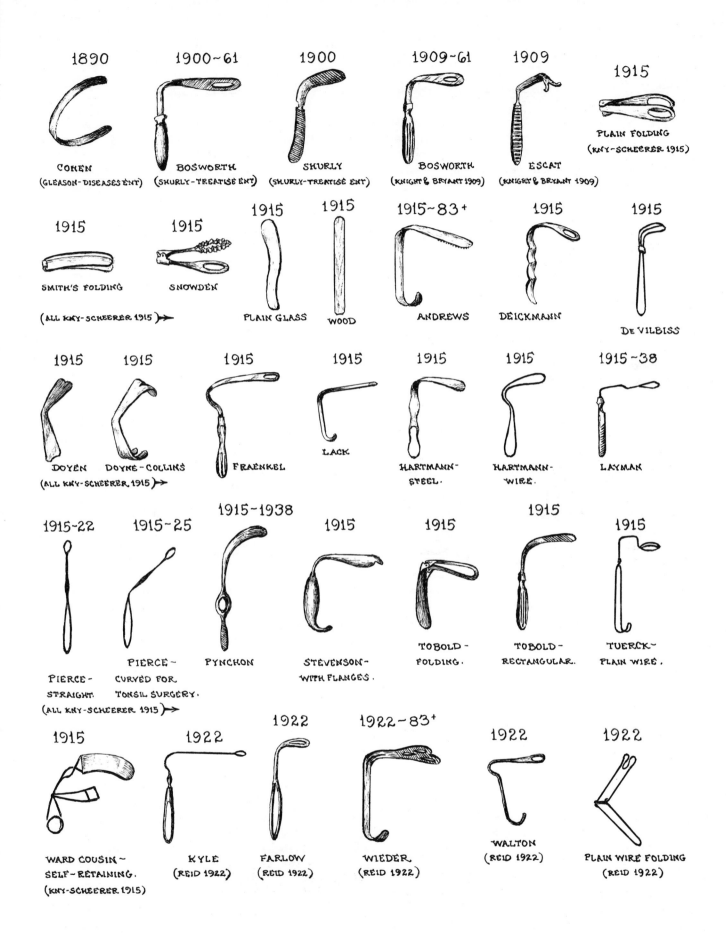

1890
COHEN
(GLEASON - DISEASES ENT)

1900~61
BOSWORTH
(SHURLY - TREATISE ENT)

1900
SHURLY
(SHURLY - TREATISE ENT)

1909~61
BOSWORTH
(KNIGHT & BRYANT 1909)

1909
ESCAT
(KNIGHT & BRYANT 1909)

1915
PLAIN FOLDING
(KNY-SCHEERER 1915)

1915
SMITH'S FOLDING
(ALL KNY-SCHEERER 1915) ➤

1915
SNOWDEN

1915
PLAIN GLASS

1915
WOOD

1915~83+
ANDREWS

1915
DEICKMANN

1915
DE VILBISS

1915
DOYEN

1915
DOYNE - COLLINS
(ALL KNY-SCHEERER 1915) ➤

1915
FRAENKEL

1915
LACK

1915
HARTMANN-STEEL.

1915
HARTMANN-WIRE.

1915~38
LAYMAN

1915~22
PIERCE-STRAIGHT.
(ALL KNY-SCHEERER 1915) ➤

1915~25
PIERCE-CURVED FOR TONSIL SURGERY.

1915~1938
PYNCHON

1915
STEVENSON-WITH FLANGES.

1915
TOBOLD-FOLDING.

1915
TOBOLD-RECTANGULAR.

1915
TUERCK-PLAIN WIRE.

1915
WARD COUSIN~SELF-RETAINING.
(KNY-SCHEERER 1915)

1922
KYLE
(REID 1922)

1922
FARLOW
(REID 1922)

1922~83+
WIEDER
(REID 1922)

1922
WALTON
(REID 1922)

1922
PLAIN WIRE FOLDING
(REID 1922)

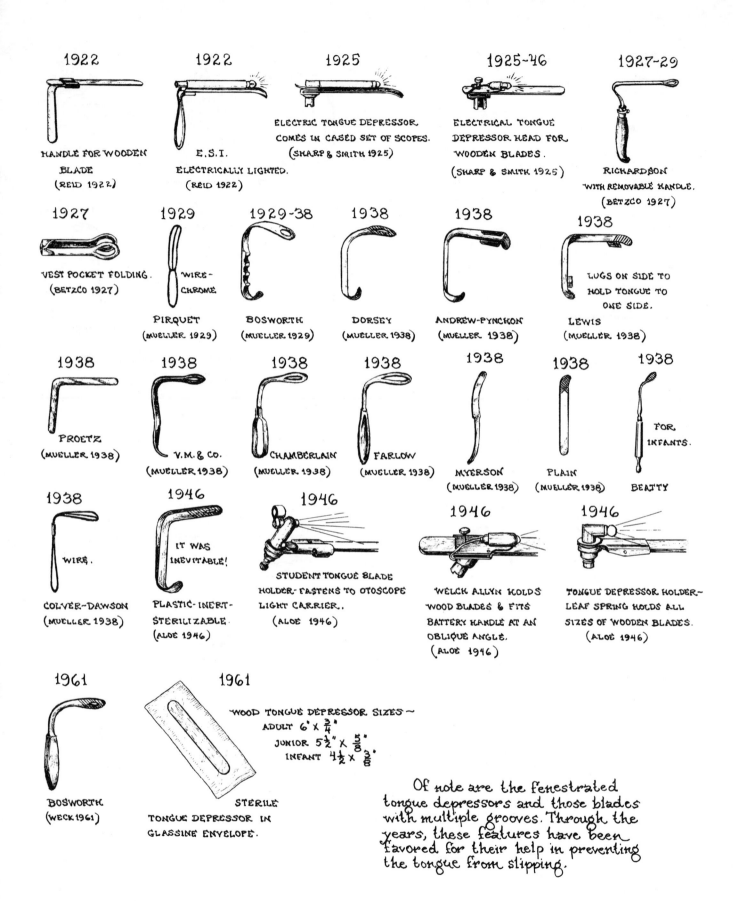

1922
HANDLE FOR WOODEN BLADE
(REID 1922)

1922
E.S.I.
ELECTRICALLY LIGHTED.
(REID 1922)

1925
ELECTRIC TONGUE DEPRESSOR.
COMES IN CASED SET OF SCOPES.
(SHARP & SMITH 1925)

1925-46
ELECTRICAL TONGUE DEPRESSOR HEAD FOR WOODEN BLADES.
(SHARP & SMITH 1925)

1927-29
RICHARDSON WITH REMOVABLE HANDLE.
(BETZCO 1927)

1927
VEST POCKET FOLDING.
(BETZCO 1927)

1929
WIRE-CHROME
PIRQUET
(MUELLER 1929)

1929-38
BOSWORTH
(MUELLER 1929)

1938
DORSEY
(MUELLER 1938)

1938
ANDREW-PYNCHON
(MUELLER 1938)

1938
LUGS ON SIDE TO HOLD TONGUE TO ONE SIDE.
LEWIS
(MUELLER 1938)

1938
PROETZ
(MUELLER 1938)

1938
V.M. & CO.
(MUELLER 1938)

1938
CHAMBERLAIN
(MUELLER 1938)

1938
FARLOW
(MUELLER 1938)

1938
MYERSON
(MUELLER 1938)

1938
PLAIN
(MUELLER 1938)

1938
FOR INFANTS.
BEATTY

1938
WIRE.
COLVER-DAWSON
(MUELLER 1938)

1946
IT WAS INEVITABLE!
PLASTIC-INERT-STERILIZABLE.
(ALOE 1946)

1946
STUDENT TONGUE BLADE HOLDER-FASTENS TO OTOSCOPE LIGHT CARRIER.
(ALOE 1946)

1946
WELCH ALLYN HOLDS WOOD BLADES & FITS BATTERY HANDLE AT AN OBLIQUE ANGLE.
(ALOE 1946)

1946
TONGUE DEPRESSOR HOLDER- LEAF SPRING HOLDS ALL SIZES OF WOODEN BLADES.
(ALOE 1946)

1961
BOSWORTH
(WECK 1961)

1961
STERILE TONGUE DEPRESSOR IN GLASSINE ENVELOPE.

WOOD TONGUE DEPRESSOR SIZES ~
ADULT 6" X ¾"
JUNIOR 5½" X ⁹⁄₁₆"
INFANT 4½ X ³⁄₈"

Of note are the fenestrated tongue depressors and those blades with multiple grooves. Through the years, these features have been favored for their help in preventing the tongue from slipping.

ENDOSCOPES

THE LARYNGOSCOPE

The reflecting hand mirror and the later head lamp cleared the darkness from many of the bodily openings. There was still the matter of just what lay around the bend of that opening. As for the larynx, the early nineteeth century physician might just as well tried exploring the twistings and turnings of a cave without benefit of candle. An endoscope was needed~defined by Webster as "an instrument for examining the interior of a bodily canal or hollow organ." Any such early diagnostic tool would require both illumination and light reflection.

In 1805, Philipp Bozzini of Frankfort developed an idea that became the prototype for much later endoscopes. Inside a tin leather-covered vase-shaped lantern was a candle. Light from an off-set polished candle holder reflected into the speculum. A horozontal partition in the speculum separated this illumination from the rays returning to the physician's eye. A lens and eyepiece at the back of the lantern enlarged the reflection from the oral cavity.

As so often happens, there was jealousy afoot in the Vienna Medical Faculty. Certainly Bozzini's instrument was found wanting in candle power, and it lacked vision beyond the pharynx. The Faculty came down heavily on these shortcomings, and the "Lichtleiter's" potential went unappreciated for almost three quarters of a century until Edison's modified electric light was better able to brighten the pharyngolaryngeal area.

Meanwhile, in 1825 Dr. Benjamin Guy Babington combined simplicity with practicality when he invented the first true laryngoscope. Were it not for the epiglottis that blocked the vocal cords from view, the "glottiscope" would have been an important addition to the doctor's bag.

1805
BOZZINI'S LICHTLEITER WITH ORAL SPECULUM.

(AMERICAN COLLEGE OF SURGEONS)

SEE CYSTOSCOPE SECTION FOR INTERNAL SKETCHES.

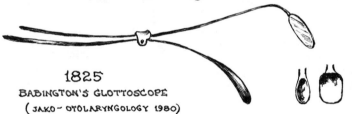

1825
BABINGTON'S GLOTTOSCOPE
(JAKO ~ OTOLARYNGOLOGY 1980)

A LARYNGEAL MIRROR AND TONGUE DEPRESSOR WERE JOINED BY A SPRING. WHEN THE TWO HANDLES WERE PRESSED TOGETHER, THE TONGUE WAS DEPRESSED. WITH THE PATIENT'S BACK TO THE SUN, DR. BABINGTON REFLECTED LIGHT ONTO THE LARYNGEAL MIRROR WITH AN ORDINARY HAND MIRROR. (LATER PHYSICIANS WOULD THEN USE A HEAD MIRROR INSTEAD OF ONE THAT WAS HAND-HELD ~ A FAR EASIER PROCEDURE)

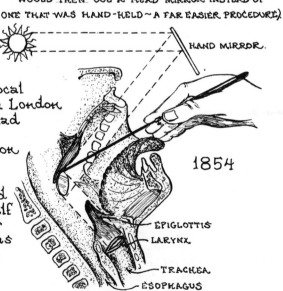

HAND MIRROR.

Although out of sight, the larynx was certainly not out of mind. In 1854, the first really workable laryngoscope and the study of the vocal cords came from an unlikely source~a London singing master. M. Manuel Garcia had long toyed with the idea that the larynx might be seen with a common dental mirror~in use for such as scaling for centuries. When on vacation in Paris, the distinguished teacher experimented upon himself with just such a small mirror on a long bent stem. This was placed against the uvula~his

1833
DENTAL MIRROR
BY
JOHN D. CHEVALIER,
NEW YORK CITY.
MOTHER-OF-PEARL.

(WEINBERGER~INTRODUCTION HISTORY DENTISTRY.)

1854

EPIGLOTTIS
LARYNX
TRACHEA
ESOPHAGUS

gag reflex may have also been on vacation~ and a second hand-held mirror directed the sun's rays onto the laryngeal mirror. The vocal cords were clearly reflected. His paper, presented to the Royal Society of London, gave the first account of the larynx during inspiration and vocalization. Still, the laryngoscope was hardly ready for office diagnosis.

Professor Czermak of Pesth brought practicality to the effort in 1857. First, he replaced the unpredictable sunlight with artificial lamp light. He then modified the perforated concave ophthalmic mirror of Ruete into the first reflecting head mirror. An 1858 photo also showed the professor with what appeared to be a mouth-held mirror before his eye. Like Garcia, Czermak practiced on his own larynx, (it is said that he was blessed with a cavernous pharynx, tiny tonsils and uvula, and sizable vocal cords). His enthusiastic writings and demonstrations brought wide acceptance of the basic laryngoscope that continues in use today.

Until then, America was underwhelmed by the many indirect laryngoscopy efforts. Now proven and practical, Louis Elsberg brought the concept home to New York City in 1861. Meanwhile, Boston practitioner Ephraim Cutter visited Czermak at Paris in 1856, and then had a tinsmith fashion his own set of laryngoscopic mirrors. With them he was even able to photograph his own larynx five years later. His crusade to popularize the new technique was well received~although his own medical school, Harvard, did not introduce laryngoscopy into its curriculum until 1875.

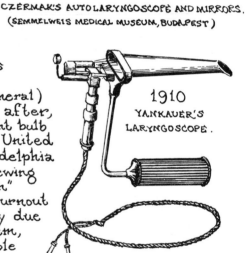

1858
CZERMAK'S AUTOLARYNGOSCOPE AND MIRRORS.
(SEMMELWEIS MEDICAL MUSEUM, BUDAPEST)

With the invention of Edison's incandescent bulb in 1879, DIRECT laryngoscopy (and endoscopes in general) became a very real possibility. Soon after, Max Nitze pioneered a miniature light bulb and a distally~lit cystoscope. In the United States, Chevalier Jackson of Philadelphia modified the idea into a direct viewing laryngoscope. A distal "wheat grain" bulb lit the field~sometimes. Quick burnout as well as minimal illumination, partly due to the light absorption by the concave lens system, did not hide the fact that here was an admirable diagnostic tool. This was confirmed as new improvements made it all the more useful.

1895
KIRSTEIN'S DIRECT LARYNGOSCOPE.

1910
YANKAUER'S LARYNGOSCOPE.

FOR BINOCULAR VIEWING.

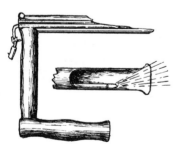

1902
CHEVALIER JACKSON'S
DETACHABLE HANDLE USED FOR SITTING
PATIENTS OR WHEN HELD BY ASSISTANT.
(KNIGHT & BRYANT-DISEASES ENT 1909)

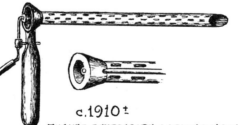

c.1910±
TUCKER RETROGRADE LARYNGOSCOPE
GABRIEL TUCKER, M.D. OF PHILADELPHIA
WAS AN ASSOCIATE OF CHEVALIER
JACKSON.
(MUTTER MUSEUM, PHILADELPHIA.)

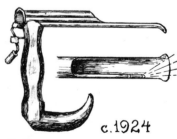

c.1924
IMPROVED JACKSON'S MODEL
(SHARP & SMITH CO. 1925)

THE MID-TWENTIES PRODUCED A
NUMBER OF VARIATIONS TO THE
JACKSON~ALL SIMILAR.

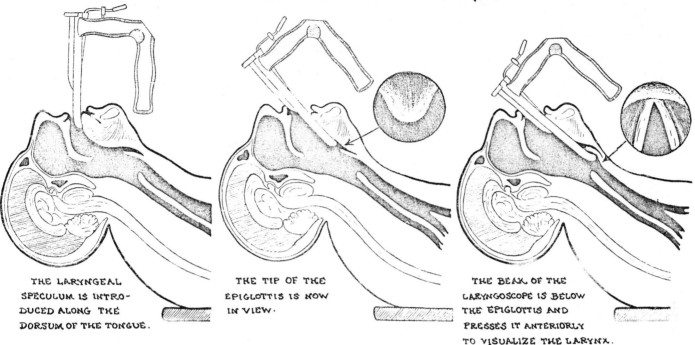

THE LARYNGEAL SPECULUM IS INTRO-DUCED ALONG THE DORSUM OF THE TONGUE.

THE TIP OF THE EPIGLOTTIS IS NOW IN VIEW.

THE BEAK OF THE LARYNGOSCOPE IS BELOW THE EPIGLOTTIS AND PRESSES IT ANTERIORLY TO VISUALIZE THE LARYNX.

(ILLUSTRATIONS FROM IMPERATORI AND BURMAN~DISEASES OF THE NOSE AND THROAT 1939)

In 1930, Lamm introduced the revolutionary fiberoptic concept. High optical density glass fibers were coated with a lower optical density glass. Once formed in a bundle, these fibers not only transmitted a brilliant light for viewing, but also returned a sharp image to the viewer. The bundle could be bent into a complete circle without decreasing light or distorting the image ~ and there were no problem prisms or lenses as in the past. In addition, viewing the larynx by the nasal route needed no traumatic rigid nasopharyngo-laryngoscope by 1975.

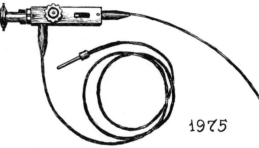

1975

THE FIRST PRACTICAL NASOPHARYNGOLARYNGOSCOPE. IT WEIGHED 0.2 KG. and was 25 cm. long EXCLUDING THE CONTROL SECTION.

(SILBERMAN ~ MEDICAL TIMES, MARCH 1982)

The new fiberoptic scope weighed but six ounces (0.2 kg.) and its diameter of less than four milimeters passed easily through the nasal cavities.

Dr. Harvey Silberman notes in the "Medical Times" of March 1982 that "Another important advancement was the recent introduction of the telescopic rod system by Hopkins. This innovation cleverly reverses the glass~to~air relationship within an endoscopic telescope. Air is used as the lens, with interspersed glass rods having concave polished ends. The light is transmitted by fiberoptics, and because of the unique lens system, very little light is absorbed by the lens system, which results in a brighter image."

BRONCHOSCOPES

1898
KILLIAN'S BRONCHOSCOPE OR ESOPHAGOSCOPE
9 mm. DIAMETER ~ 18, 28, 35 AND 41 CM. IN LENGTH.
(KNY-SCHEERER 1915)

Beyond the larynx, the bronchi had long been trouble spots for inhaled foreign bodies. Killian introduced his solution to this problem in 1898 ~ the first rigid bronchoscope. This simple tube not only was useful for removing these obstructions, but also proved a valuable diagnostic tool as well.

Four years later, Dr. Chevalier Jackson of Philadelphia had improved the device and then added grasping and biopsy instruments. Any doubts about the new bronchoscope were laid to rest when his timeless 1907 text on the technique of bronchoscopy was published. To prevent encroachment on the tiny lumen (a nine centimeter diameter was about all the bronchial tubes could handle) the light carrier channel was either part of the tube wall or attached to its outer wall. Aspirating channels were added later ~ a compromise between keeping the field clear of secretions and further decreasing the diameter of the lumen.

1902
JACKSON'S BRONCHOSCOPE ~
SLANTED END MADE INTRODUCTION EASIER.
(KNIGHT & BRYANT ~ DISEASES OF N.T. + E. 1909)

1920's
JACKSON'S ASPIRATING BRONCHOSCOPE
5, 6, 7, 8 mm DIAMETERS AND 30, 40, 45, 4 cm.
LENGTHS. (MUELLER & CO. 1929)

Through the years, Jackson's bronchoscope was the standard against which all others were compared. Several early "others" include:

HOLINGER BRONCHOSCOPE.
(MUTTER MUSEUM, PHILADELPHIA.)

TUCKER INFANT BRONCHOSCOPE
(MUTTER MUSEUM, PHILADELPHIA.)

Rigid bronchoscopy requires a local anesthetic to the upper airways, although a general anesthetic is sometimes used for children and apprehensive adults. With the patient lying down and the head fully extended, the bronchoscope is passed directly into the trachea and bronchi. Rigid bronchoscopy has not been entirely elbowed aside by the bronchofiberscope. Indeed, it is still preferred for removing foreign bodies from the respiratory tree, as well as use in small children, packing areas of heavy bleeding, or excising vascular lesions as adenomas or granulation tissue.

THE ADULT 'SCOPE USED IS GENERALLY 7 mm. BY 40 cm.

The fiberoptic concept reached the bronchial passages in 1970, and American physicians responded with an enthusiasm that continues today. Thin and flexible, its directional control at the tip gives easier passage into the subsegmental bronchi for both diagnosis and treatment. A set of objectives and oculars at either end of the glass fibers bring any pathology into sharp focus.

The nasal route is preferred after premedication and local lidocaine. Lidocaine is also passed through the inner channel of the bronchofiberscope to anesthetize the bronchi. It should be noted that this very narrow channel will not provide adequate lung ventilation unless oxygen is administered. The patient is usually lying down although the patient may also be seated and facing the physician.

PENTAX AD | ©1982

THE GASTROSCOPE

Quite by accident~ a discharged musket, actually~ the secrets of gastric physiology were discovered. It was in June of 1822, and the unlikely laboratory was the frontier American fort at Mackinac. A French Canadian voyageur, Alexis St. Martin, had sustained a close range blast that penetrated the left lower lung and stomach. Dr William Beaumont, a young army physician stationed at the outpost, managed to bring his new patient back to health~ but with a permanent gastric fistula[1].

Beaumont, while supporting and caring for the fellow under his own roof, realized that the functionings of the stomach could be studied directly. From these observations, as summarized by Osler, came our knowledge of the gastric juices, importance of hydrochloric acid, the effect of mental stress on acid secretion and digestion, comparative studies on digestion inside and outside the stomach, correction of many myths about stomach function, the digestibility of various foods, and the first comprehensive study of the motility of the stomach.

With the exception of his gastric fistula, there was little that was admirable about St. Martin. Cantankerous, unpredictable and untrustworthy, it was in spite of and not because of him that Dr. Beaumont succeeded in his investigations. Throughout the world, fellow physicians learned of his discoveries through his Experiments and Observations... in 1833. Reprints followed in 1834 and 1847, as well as a German translation in 1834 and a Scottish edition in 1838.

With interest focused on the workings of the stomach, John Hunter invented the stomach tube in England and Philip Syng Physick brought the instrument to America. Unfortunately, intubation received little notice until 1867, when Kussmaul performed a gastric lavage[2] on a twenty year old country girl with a pyloric stricture[3]. Pumped free of three liters of acid and undigested food, it was clear that vomiting was no longer the preferred way to rid the stomach of unwanted contents. The technique quickly became an accepted treatment, and with it the possibilities for diagnosis. By the first decade of the twentieth century, routine gastric analysis and diagnosis of aspirated cancer cells had become a reality.

FOR 7 YEARS, BEAUMONT EXPERIMENTED ON GASTRIC FUNCTIONS THROUGH ST. MARTIN'S FISTULA.

"NOW A FELLOW MAY ENJOY HIMSELF BY EATING THREE DINNERS". AN EARLY NINETEENTH CENTURY CARTOON LAMPOONING THE STOMACH PUMP.

STOMACH TUBES
(REKFUSS~DISEASES OF THE STOMACH, 1927)

[1] AN ABNORMAL STOMACH PASSAGE.   [2] WASHING OUT THE STOMACH.   [3] A CONSTRICTED LOWER STOMACH.

Introduction of a gastroscope had a near miss in 1848 after Dr. Campbell of Glasgow watched a sword swallower at a country fair. But when the performer saw Campbell's long round tube, he protested "I know I can swallow a sword, but I'll be —— if I can swallow a trumpet!" Perhaps it would have proved an exercise in futility. Prior to the invention of electricity and the miniature light bulb, the gastroscope was impractical. Chevalier Jackson was, however, remarkably adept at passing the tube into the stomach in spite of a very limited visual field.

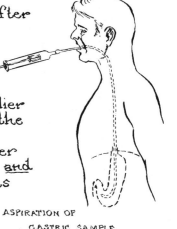

ASPIRATION OF GASTRIC SAMPLE.

By 1911, the gastroscope came into its own when Elsner passed a rigid tube that was outfitted with mirrors, prisms and that all important distal "grain of wheat" bulb. Many such efforts followed — and many with unhappy results. Esophageal injury, pressure necrosis and even perforation were a very real danger.

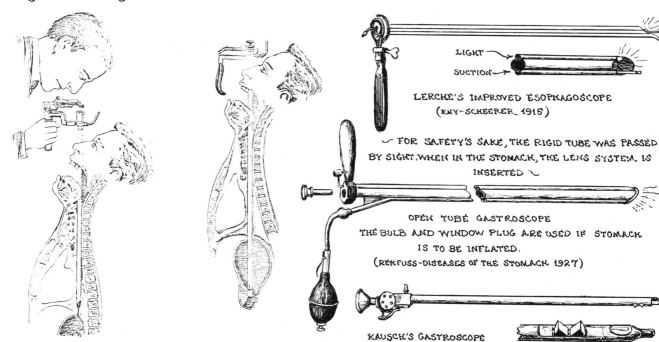

ESOPHAGOSCOPE   GASTROSCOPE
(ILLUSTRATION FROM AARON-DISEASES OF THE DIGESTIVE ORGANS 1921)

LIGHT
SUCTION

LERCHE'S IMPROVED ESOPHAGOSCOPE
(KNY-SCHEERER 1915)

~ FOR SAFETY'S SAKE, THE RIGID TUBE WAS PASSED BY SIGHT. WHEN IN THE STOMACH, THE LENS SYSTEM IS INSERTED ᴗ

OPEN TUBE GASTROSCOPE
THE BULB AND WINDOW PLUG ARE USED IF STOMACH IS TO BE INFLATED.
(REKFUSS-DISEASES OF THE STOMACH 1927)

KAUSCH'S GASTROSCOPE
LENS SYSTEM IS FLAT WHEN PASSED, THEN MAY BE ANGLED INTO POSITION TO VIEW STOMACH WALLS.
(MUELLER & CO. 1929)

Mindful of such hazards, Rudolph Schindler worked with the optical firm of G. Wolf to produce the first working flexible gastroscope. His successful demonstration of the instrument in 1932 opened a new endoscopic era. The old rigid tube was obsolete. It was America's good fortune that Schindler emigrated to the United States in 1934, spreading the word of his new instrument and the necessary technique.

Hirschowitz followed up with the first fully flexible fiberoptic gastroscope in 1958. Improvements came rapidly, for the diameters of gastroscopes were decreased and the optical systems were further perfected. Gastroscope tips could now have full end flexion with controlling wires. Accessory channels permit suction, insufflation of air and passage of biopsy forceps, cytology brushes and snares — an all purpose instrument.

① LOCALIZED DEATH OF LIVING TISSUE FROM GASTROSCOPIC PRESSURE.

VAGINAL SPECULA

Since therapy prior to 1800 was based on symptoms and not physical findings, there was little need for diagnostic instruments. The vaginal specula were one notable exception, and the French surgeon Jacques Dalechamps (1512-1588) went so far as to say that these instruments were in common use. Indeed, the Greeks and Romans made mention of such specula, and bivalve, trivalve and quadravalve specula were excavated at Pompeii. It is also possible that simple cylinders had seen service during those early years. All in all, the large and formidable three-bladed turn-screw speculum was most favored.

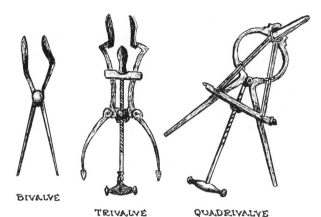

BIVALVE

TRIVALVE   QUADRIVALVE

VAGINAL SPECULA FOUND AT POMPEII.
THE SCREW FORCED THE UPPER BLADES OUTWARD.

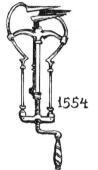

1554

RUEFF SPECULUM.
(DE CONCEPTU ET
GENEATIONE HOMINIS...
RUEFF, ZURICH 1554)

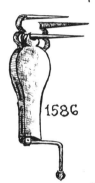

1586

AMBROISE PARÉ
(GYNAECIORUM PHYSICUS
ET CHIRURGICUS
BAUHIN, BASEL, 1586)

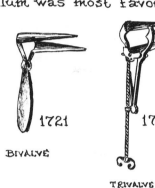

1721

BIVALVE

1721

TRIVALVE
(BIBLIOTHECA CHIRURGICA, VOL II
MANGET, GENEVA 1721)

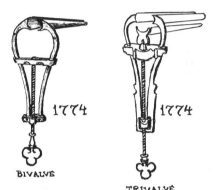

1774

BIVALVE

1774

TRIVALVE

JEAN LOUIS PETIT
(TRAITÉ DES MALADIES CHIRURGICAL,
PETIT, PARIS, 1774)

The pre-nineteenth century patient was examined while lying on her back in a chair in the knee-chest position. The closed and well-oiled blades were inverted and held in place by the physician. An assistant turned the upright handle "softly without violence" to expand the blades.

Early America seems to have completely ignored the speculum. Perhaps this was because obstetrics (and its related anatomy) was beneath the dignity and modesty of the few practicing physicians. Meanwhile, midwives went about the business of bringing new colonists into the world, and fancy European gadgets were quite beyond their expertise.

CYLINDRICAL SPECULA ~ Such was the state of affairs until an old idea was reconsidered in 1801. Joseph Récamier, considered by many as the first gynocology specialist, needed no team effort for his simple speculum. His five inch long tin tube could be easily inserted, and its shiny inner surface reflected more light to see the cervix clearly. Unfortunately, the vaginal wall was hidden when the cylinder was in place. Récamier made several alterations, including a scooped-out section for better viewing. Over the later years, the tube saw many changes, using such materials as metal, ivory, glass, porcelain, wood and India rubber.

CYLINDRICAL
SPECULUM

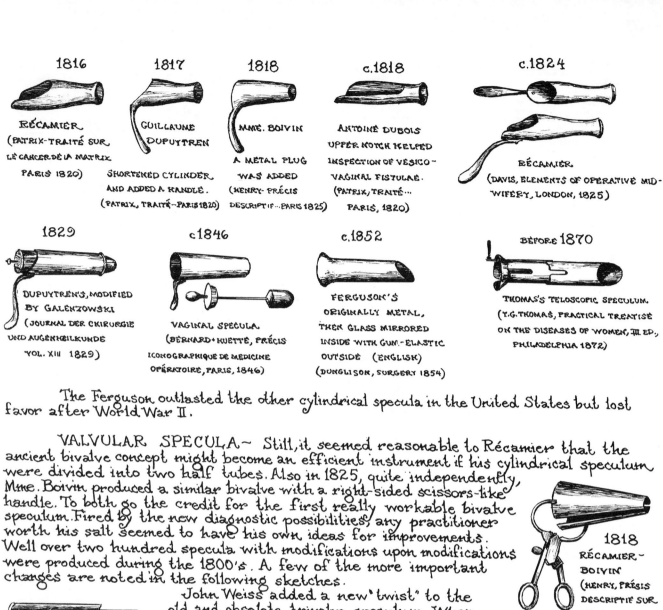

The Ferguson outlasted the other cylindrical specula in the United States but lost favor after World War II.

VALVULAR SPECULA~ Still, it seemed reasonable to Récamier that the ancient bivalve concept might become an efficient instrument if his cylindrical speculum were divided into two half tubes. Also in 1825, quite independently, Mme. Boivin produced a similar bivalve with a right-sided scissors-like handle. To both go the credit for the first really workable bivalve speculum. Fired by the new diagnostic possibilities, any practitioner worth his salt seemed to have his own ideas for improvements. Well over two hundred specula with modifications upon modifications were produced during the 1800's. A few of the more important changes are noted in the following sketches.

John Weiss added a new "twist" to the old and obsolete trivalve speculum. When closed, its narrow diameter and plug allowed for a painless introduction. A turn of the handle opened the blades for a full vaginal inspection. Actually, this bulky and expensive instrument seemed to work better for anal rather than vaginal exploration. Considerable pain was caused by the thin expanding blades, and the dullness on their inner surfaces from vaginal secretions prevented any sort of light reflection.

Actually Weiss's problems had been solved a year earlier by fellow Londoner David Davis. His four-bladed instrument did indeed prevent the mucous membrane from falling between the blades. The plug was first made of wood and later of vulcanite.

Philippe Ricord's modified speculum expanded at both ends around a fixed center joint that rested at the vaginal orifice. An oblique handle was attached to each of two blades to control expansion.

1818 RÉCAMIER-BOIVIN (HENRY, PRÉSIS DESCRIPTIF SUR LES INSTRUMENTS... PARIS, 1825)

1831 JOHN WEISS (WEISS INSTRUMENT CATALOGUE, LONDON 1831) PLUG.

1830 DAVID DAVIS (THOMPSON, THE HISTORY AND EVOLUTION OF SURGICAL INSTRUMENTS, 1942)

1834 PHILIPPE RICORD (DUNGLISON, SURGERY, 1854)

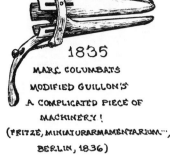

1835

MARC COLUMBATS
MODIFIED GUILLON'S
A COMPLICATED PIECE OF
MACHINERY !
(FRITZE, MINIATURARMAMENTARIUM ...,
BERLIN, 1836)

1837

JOSEPH CHARRIÈRE'S
INNOVATION HAD 3 BLADES
OVERLAPPING THE PLUG. UPON
TURNING THE SCREW, THE BLADES
UNFOLDED TO ENLARGE ITS DIAMETER.
PAUL SÉGALAS ALSO DEVELOPED A LIKE
INSTRUMENT WITH 4 BLADES.
(THOMPSON, HISTORY SURGICAL INSTRUMENTS 1942)

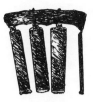

1837
BEAUMONT

THIS ENGLISH SURGEON TOOK HIS
CUE FROM HIPPOCRATIC SPECULA ITS 4 OR
5 STEEL BLADES, EACH 3 INCHES LONG,
WERE FIXED TO A METAL RING 1 INCH
IN DIAMETER. ACCORDING TO THOMPSON,
A SCREW IN THE RING'S CENTER WORKED
BY A HANDLE THAT PASSED INTO THE
BLADES. EACH BLADE HAD A SCREW
THAT DREW THEM TOGETHER. WITH A
STRING WHEN IN PLACE, THE BLADES
WERE EXPANDED AND THE HANDLE UN-
SCREWED. CONFUSING!
(THOMPSON, HISTORY OF SURGICAL INSTRUMENTS,
1941)

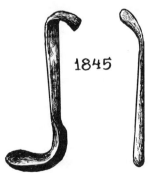

c.1850?
EDOUARD CUSCO
1819-1894

CUSCO'S BIVALVE WAS THE MOST
POPULAR DURING THIS EARLIER PERIOD
AND CONTINUES IN USE TO THIS DAY.
IT WAS THE FORERUNNER OF THE
GRAVES SPECULUM.
(REYNDERS CATALOGUE, NEW YORK 1895)

Cusco's blades were unique~they were indeed shaped like duck's bills and are preferred today. T. Gaillard Thomas, in his <u>Diseases of Women</u> (1872) states that "Of valvular specula the bivalve of Ricord, the trivalve of Ségalas, and the quadrivalve of Charrière have long been popular [in America]. No instrument of this variety with which I am acquainted equals in beauty and utility that of M. Cusco. It is compact, easily introduced, and shows the cervix very clearly." He went on to say that the introduction of these bladed instruments caused much less pain than the cylindrical specula. However, prolapse of the vaginal wall between the blades was a disadvantage, as well as possible pinching when the instrument was removed. Probing of the uterus or applications to the fundus was difficult. "Sims' speculum, which is in reality a bivalve, obviates all these difficulties in a most complete and satisfactory manner."

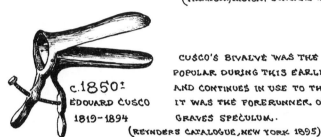

1845

SIMS' ORIGINAL VAGINAL
SPECULUM AND A SPATULA
USED TO PRESS THE URETHRA
AGAINST THE SYMPHYSIS FOR
FISTULA REPAIR.
(AMERICAN JOURNAL OF MEDICAL
SCIENCES, VOL. XXIII 1852)

LATER VERSION OF SIMS'
SPECULUM WITH DUCK-BILL
BLADES AND DEPRESSOR.
(T.G. THOMAS, DISEASES OF
WOMEN, PHILADELPHIA, 1872)

Sims' instrument was born of the American make-do-or-do-without tradition. Having forgotten his old speculum while on a distant house call, Dr. Sims stopped at a general store and purchased a pewter spoon. He bent each end at opposing right angles, and found his makeshift speculum worked well indeed.

Sims found his speculum most useful in exposing vesico-vaginal fistulae ~ and later making surgical history with his successful repair of the problem. It was not until some time after 1852 that the familiar speculum with two "duck~bill" blades came into being.

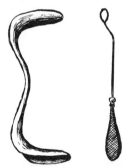

SIMS' POSITION

The usual position of the patient was still knee-chest. Sims, after 1852, found that if the patient were in the left lateral position, air would distend the entire vaginal passage when his speculum lifted the posterior vaginal wall. A landmark for diagnosis and surgery!

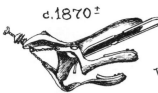

c.1870±

NOTT'S SPECULUM OPEN
(THOMAS, DISEASES OF
WOMEN 1872)

An assistant was needed to hold the Sims' speculum. Dr. Nott's device converted the examination into a one man procedure with its two short arms pressing securely against the anterior vaginal wall.

The important Graves' speculum was invented by Dr. T.W. Graves, a general practitioner from Woburn, Massachusetts. The lower blade retracted the posterior vaginal wall while the sliding bar handle pressed the anterior blade under the pubic arch. It was then secured in position by the set screw and no assistant was necessary. It remains the most popular American vaginal speculum today.

Using John Reynder's New York catalogue of 1895 for an end-of-the century comparison, one may have an idea of other speculum popularity spans.

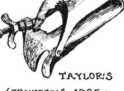
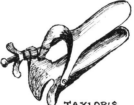

1878
GRAVES SPECULUM.

(REYNDER'S CATALOGUE, 1895)

GRAVES' REVERSIBLE TO SIMS' SPECULUM..

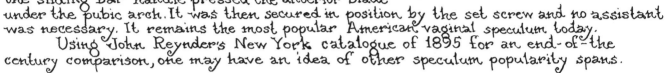

1895~1930	1895~1940	1895~1940	1895~1965

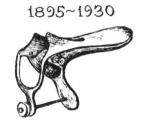

BREWER'S
(REYNDER'S 1895 –
MAKADY CO. 1929)

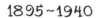
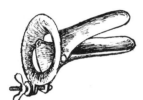

HIGBEE'S
(REYNDER'S 1895~
V.MUELLER CO. 1938)

TAYLOR'S
(REYNDER'S 1895 –
V. MUELLER CO. 1938)

MILLER'S
(REYNDER'S 1895 –
WECK CO. 1961)

1895~1930	1895~1925	1895~1975+	1915~1975+	1915~1981+

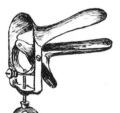
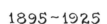
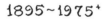

HALES
(REYNDER'S 1895 –
MAKADY CO. 1929)

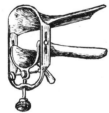

JACKSON'S
(REYNDER'S 1895 –
SHARP & SMITH 1925)

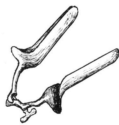

COLLIN'S
(REYNDER'S 1895~
MILTEX 1973)

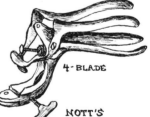

4-BLADE

NOTT'S
(REID 1915 –
MILTEX 1973)

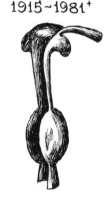

AUVARD'S
(REID 1915 – WECK & CO. 1982)

1929~1982+

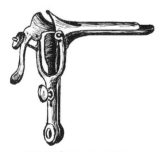

PEDERSON~GRAVES
WECK/SCHEIN 1981+

LIFE SPAN OF THOSE SPECULA NOTED IN TEXT:
FERGUSON'S CYLINDRICAL c1852~1925 (DUNGLISON, 1854~SHARP & SMITH 1925)
RICORD'S BIVALVE 1834~1880± (DUNGLISON 1854~THOMAS, DISEASES OF WOMEN 1872)
SÉGALAS TRIVALVE c1837 TO 1880± (THOMAS 1872)
CHARRIÈRE'S QUADRIVALVE 1837~1880± (THOMAS 1872~RICCI, DEVEL.GYN. INSTRUMENTS 1949)
CUSCO'S BIVALVE c.1850±~1980+ (RICCI, DEVEL. GYN. INSTRUMENTS 1949~MILTEX CO. 1973)
SIMS' 1845~1982+ (AMERICAN JOURNAL MED. SCIENCES 1852~WECK CO. 1982)
NOTT'S QUADRIVALVE c1870~1965 (THOMAS 1872~WECK 1961)
GRAVES BIVALVE 1878~1983+ (RICCI 1949~SCHEIN CO. 1983)

RECTAL INSTRUMENTS

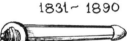

While the rectum has never been a topic for polite conversation, it continues to be the "butt" of jokesters. "Joe had constipation and the Doc checked him out with a long tube." "Rectum?" "Rectum~darn near killed'um!" It's that part of the anatomy especially designed for annoying itching and painful fissures, fistulas and hemorrhoids. It's been the object of the frantic colonic irrigations that gushed through the eighteenth and nineteenth centuries here and abroad~including the prim and proper Victorian days. Frequently, past patients and their physicians have opted for suppositories rather than a search for a possible obstructing cancer.

Hippocrates and other Greek healers were familiar with the two~bladed rectal speculum~used also for vaginal examination. But its use had little emphasis until 1835. It was then that Frederick Salmon of London founded THE INFIRMARY FOR THE RELIEF OF THE POOR AFFLICTED WITH FISTULA AND OTHER DISEASES OF THE RECTUM. It was as long a name as it was short on sympathy from fellow physicians. Yet Dr. Salmon's one man crusade had proved its value. When he retired in 1859, he had operated on 3500 patients without a fatality.

BIVALVE RECTAL AND VAGINAL SPECULUM FOUND IN POMPEII.

Perhaps the Infirmary used a speculum much like the ancient rectal bivalve, or the newer Weiss narrow cylinder bivalve or the fenestrated cone.

1666~1721

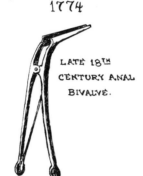

BIVALVE ANAL SPECULUM~ LITTLE CHANGED FROM GRECIAN DAYS.

(CULTETUS ARMAMENTARIUM CHIRURGICUM, FRANKFORT, 1666 AND MANGET, BIBLIOTHECA CHIRURGICA, GENEVA., VOL. II, 1721

1774

LATE 18TH CENTURY ANAL BIVALVE.

(PETITE, TRAITÉ DES MALADIES CHIRURGICAL, PARIS, 1774)

1782

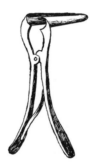

(BRAMBILLA, INSTRUMENTARIUM MILITARE AUSTRIACUM, VIENNA. 1782)

1831~ 1890

'WEISS' RECTAL (AND VAGINAL) SPECULUM.

NARROW CYLINDER TYPE.

(JOHN WEISS CATALOGUE LONDON, 1831 ~ REYNDERS, 1895)

c 1850~1862

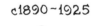

UNFORTUNATELY, THE MUCOUS MEMBRANE CAUGHT IN THE BLADES.

(DUNGLISON 1854 ~ GROSS, SYSTEM OF SURGERY, VOL.II. 1862)

c.1852~1915±

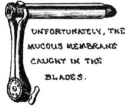

FERGUSON'S (DUNGLISON 1854)

c 1854~1862

~FENESTRATED~

(DUNGLISON 1854 ~ GROSS, SYSTEM OF SURGERY VOL II. 1862)

c1854-1915

(DUNGLISON 1854 ~ KNY-SCHEERER 1915)

c1890~1925

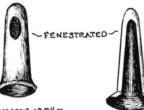

THE CONE SPECULA WERE LITTLE USED IN THE UNITED STATES AFTER WORLD WAR I.

ALLINGHAM'S (KNY-1915 ~ SHARP & SMITH 1925)

Salmon's infirmary was also known by the less exhausting title of St. Mark's Hospital. After a new enlarged building and several energetic successors, a number of post-Civil War American physicians studied at the institution. Among them, in 1877, was Dr. Joseph M. Mathews of Louisville, Kentucky~soon to become a pioneer rectal specialist here. He published the first American textbook on the subject in 1893~ <u>Treatise On Diseases of the Rectum, Anus and Sigmoid Flexure</u> and became the first president of the American Proctologic Society, founded in 1899. The following are specula used in his time and thereafter.

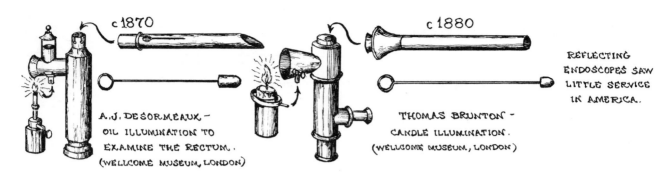

c 1870

A.J. DESORMEAUX –
OIL ILLUMINATION TO
EXAMINE THE RECTUM.
(WELLCOME MUSEUM, LONDON)

c 1880

THOMAS BRUNTON –
CANDLE ILLUMINATION.
(WELLCOME MUSEUM, LONDON)

REFLECTING
ENDOSCOPES SAW
LITTLE SERVICE
IN AMERICA.

c 1875 ~ 1880

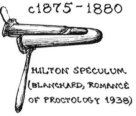

HILTON SPECULUM
(BLANCHARD, ROMANCE
OF PROCTOLOGY 1938)

DR. CHARLES BLANCHARD'S PROVOCATIVE BOOK TITLE
THE ROMANCE OF PROCTOLOGY MADE IT A MUST READING. INSIDE
THIS 1938 VOLUME HE STATES IN HIS CHATTY STYLE THAT THE
MOST USEFUL ANAL SPECULUM EVER INVENTED WAS THAT OF
JOHN HILTON. BRINKERHOFF PRESENTED AN IMPROVED VERSION
IN 1880 THAT BEARS HIS NAME. THE ROUNDED END WAS EASILY
INTRODUCED, AND THE SLIDING BLADE GAVE FULL VIEW OF SUCH
AS CRYPTS AND POLYPS. IF INTERNAL HEMORRHOIDS WERE PRESENT,
HOWEVER, IT MUST BE TILTED DOWNWARD TO PREVENT DRAGGING DOWN THE MASS.

1880 ~ 1961

BRINKERHOFF'S –
WITH LIGHT CARRIER.
(KNY-SCHEERER 1915 ~
WECK 1961)

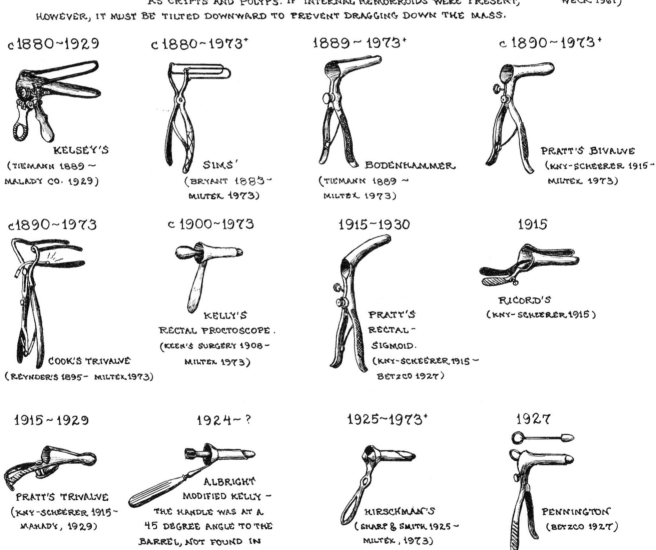

c 1880 ~ 1929

KELSEY'S
(TIEMANN 1889 ~
MALADY CO. 1929)

c 1880 ~ 1973+

SIMS'
(BRYANT 1885 ~
MILTEX 1973)

1889 ~ 1973+

BODENHAMMER
(TIEMANN 1889 ~
MILTEX 1973)

c 1890 ~ 1973+

PRATT'S BIVALVE
(KNY-SCHEERER 1915 ~
MILTEX 1973)

c 1890 ~ 1973

COOK'S TRIVALVE
(REYNDER'S 1895 ~ MILTEX 1973)

c 1900 ~ 1973

KELLY'S
RECTAL PROCTOSCOPE.
(KEEN'S SURGERY 1908 –
MILTEX 1973)

1915 ~ 1930

PRATT'S
RECTAL –
SIGMOID.
(KNY-SCHEERER 1915 ~
BETZCO 1927)

1915

RICORD'S
(KNY-SCHEERER 1915)

1915 ~ 1929

PRATT'S TRIVALVE
(KNY-SCHEERER 1915 ~
MAHADY, 1929)

1924 ~ ?

ALBRIGHT
MODIFIED KELLY –
THE HANDLE WAS AT A
45 DEGREE ANGLE TO THE
BARREL, NOT FOUND IN
CATALOGUES THEREAFTER.
(BLANCHARD, ROMANCE PROCTOLOGY 1938)

1925 ~ 1973+

HIRSCHMAN'S
(SHARP & SMITH 1925 ~
MILTEX, 1973)

1927

PENNINGTON
(BETZCO 1927)

1946~1973+

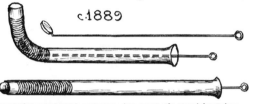

The anoscope, of course, was used for examining the anus or outlet, while the proctoscope (Greek próktos = anus) did service in the rectum. For practical purposes, the preceeding instruments served both functions. The sigmoidoscope (Greek sigmoeidēs = sigma Σ or the English "S") because it was originally a rigid tube, could only penetrate into the nearest portion of this "S" shaped part of the colon. In 1976, the 60 cm. flexible sigmoidoscope was introduced to American physicians. Its four-way tip deflection could snake the head through the sigmoid twists and even beyond into the transverse colon. With it, biopsy - and even photography are possible.

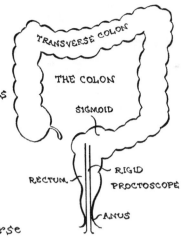

TRANSVERSE COLON
THE COLON
SIGMOID
RECTUM
RIGID PROCTOSCOPE
ANUS

BARR
SELF-RETAINING.
(ALOE 1946 ~ MILTEX 1973)

c.1889

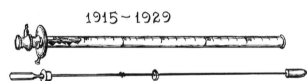

BODENHAMER'S RECTO-COLONIC ENDOSCOPE -
AN EARLY ATTEMPT WITH MIRROR REFLECTION.
(TIEMANN 1890)

1908~1973

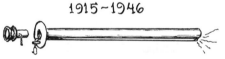

KELLY SIGMOIDOSCOPE

(KEEN, SURGERY 1908 -
MILTEX 1973)

1925 SET =
SPHINCTEROSCOPE - 2"
PROCTOSCOPE - 5½"
PROCTOSCOPE - 8"
SIGMOIDOSCOPE - 17"

1915~1929

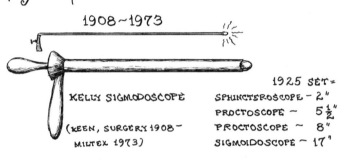

LYNCH'S PROCTO-SIGMOIDOSCOPE, OBTURATOR AND LIGHT.
(REID BROS 1915 ~ MAHADY CO. 1929)

1915~1946

TUTTLE'S PNEUMATIC PROCTO-SIGMOIDOSCOPE -
OBTURATOR, INTERCHANGEABLE WINDOW AND
LIGHT CARRIER, DETACHABLE HANDLE.
(REID BROS. 1915 ~ ALOE 1946)

1925

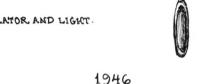

MARTIN-HIRSCHMAN'S
(SHARP & SMITH 1925)

1946

MONTAGUE SIGMOIDOSCOPE.
WELCH-ALLYN.
(ALOE 1946)

1973

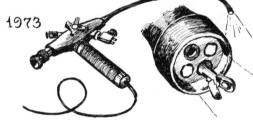

FLEXIBLE FIBER OPTIC PROCTOSIGMOIDOSCOPE
(AMERICAN OPTICAL ADVERTIZEMENT 1983)

POSITIONING THE PATIENT

THE LITHOTOMY POSITION (BELOW), ALTHOUGH COMFORTABLE
FOR THE PATIENT, PROVED
IMPRACTICAL.
c1875

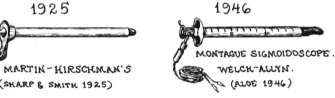

TABLE AND POSITION USED BY DR. MATHEWS.
(BLANCHARD, ROMANCE PROCTOLOGY 1938)

SIMS' POSITION (LYING ON SIDE) NEEDED
UNCOMFORTABLE INFLATION. THE DOCTOR
WAS NO BETTER OFF, FOR HIS EYE WAS
BELOW THE LEVEL OF THE SCOPE AND WAS IN
DANGER OF A DRENCHING FROM RECTAL DRAINAGE.
THE KNEE-CHEST OR KNEE-ELBOW POSITION
PROVED BEST (RIGHT) FOR THE INTESTINES FELL
DOWNWARD WITH LESS RECTAL PRESSURE. NEGATIVE
PRESSURE DISTENDED THE BOWEL WITHOUT NEED
FOR INFLATION.

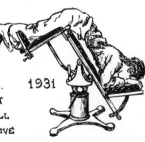

1931

(BUIE, PROCTOSCOPIC EXAM (1931)

CATHETERS (Greek kathéter = let down into or sent down)

THE RIGID CATHETER

The early Greeks recognized the diagnostic possibilities of this instrument. By exploring the urethra, stenosis (constrictions) and injury became evident. Residual bladder urine could be determined after voiding. Centuries later, it was the means for introducing contrast media into the bladder for xray diagnosis.

Excavations in Pompeii have unearthed several bronze catheters. This simple tube had changed but little until the eighteenth century. Silver, copper, brass, wax and even horn had been used, but by the early 1700's silver had won the field.

Male catheters continued the curve that better fit the urethra, but were available in various sizes. And in the 1700's the short, straight female tube became the one-size-fits-all standard. This style continued until a slight and curve became popular around 1830.

Silver plated and steel catheters began replacing the old silver tubes in the 1840's. There were those early Victorians who fancied up their new pieces with carved wooden handles. This effort died a quiet death after English surgeon Robert Liston pointed out that the sense of touch was lost when a handle was not completely smooth.

c1800
FEMALE

c1825
FEMALE

c1830
MALE

(WELLCOME MUSEUM, LONDON)

½ X

FEMALE CATHETERS

BRONZE INSTRUMENTS FOUND AT POMPEII. (VÉDRENES, TRAITÉ DE MÉDICINE... PARIS 1876)

MALE CATHETERS

c1841

NELATON'S STRAIGHT RUBBER. (LYTTON, PERSPECTIVES IN UROLOGY, VOL.I 1976)

THE FLEXIBLE CATHETER

The rigid tube had its problems, as many a distressed patient would have testified. The search was on for a catheter that would bend in the urethra's channel and not scour the mucosa in the process. There were several early efforts, among them Solingen's flexible spiral metal catheter. But the first practical breakthrough came toward the end of the eighteenth century. This French prototype of the modern gum elastic catheter was made from an ultra-secret formula. Because of it, France remained the supplier of unrivaled catheters until mid-nineteenth century innovations made important changes.

Charles Goodyear of the United States challenged this monopoly indirectly in 1839 when he successfully vulcanized crude rubber. By adding sulfa under heat and pressure, he produced a rubber that had strength, resiliency and lacked the stickiness and disagreeable odor of earlier efforts. Paris surgeon Auguste Nélaton promptly had a vulcanized catheter made for himself. The straight rubber catheter of today still bears his name.

Although the inexpensive and efficient vulcanized product had found its place in history, occasionally one would become brittle and break off in the bladder. Unfortunately, a suprapubic cystotomy was inevitable. Lewis Sayre of New Jersey and T.H. Squire of Elmira, New York independently answered the problem in 1871 by designing an articulated flexible silver catheter. The ingenious device was curved or made rigid by a threaded nut that controlled an internal chain.

Six years later, the J. Elwood Lee Company

1706

SOLINGEN'S FLEXIBLE SPIRAL CATHETER. (BENNION, ANTIQUE MED. INSTRUMENTS 1979)

c1871

SAYRE'S VERTEBRATED SILVER CATHETER (LYTTON, PERSPECTIVES IN UROLOGY VOL.I 1976)

of Conshohoken, Pennsylvania developed the prototype for today's woven nylon catheters by weaving cotton, flax and silk, and applying several layers of elasticized varnish. The more expensive had the eye woven in, while the more modest instruments had the eye punched out. It was sturdy enough to withstand repeated sterilizations in 1% carbolic acid or boiling water.

French urologist J.J. Cazenave probably had high hopes that his country would regain leadership in the catheter field. In the last of the nineteenth century, he dedicated twentyfive or thirty years of his life perfecting a flexible, durable catheter. He finally shaped and drilled ~ of all things ~ an ivory cylinder, which was then decalcified into a sort of jelly with hydrochloric acid. It was then strengthened by tanning with chlorates of lime, magnesium and ammonium salts. All this did indeed produce a workable instrument ~ quite outdated by contemporary improvements.

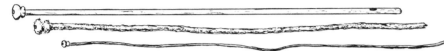

SHAPED AND DRILLED.
SOFTENED BY DECALCIFICATION.
TANNED AND DRIED ~ FINISHED.

In summary, America's late entry into the catheter field paid off handsomely with the flexible and durable vulcanized rubber and the woven catheters.

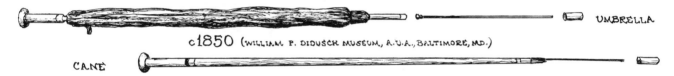

UMBRELLA

c1850 (WILLIAM P. DIDUSCH MUSEUM, A.U.A., BALTIMORE, MD.)

CANE

THESE VERY UNUSUAL FRENCH CATHETER HOLDERS FROM THE MID~1800'S SHOULD BE THE LAST WORD ON THE SUBJECT. FAIR WEATHER OR FOUL, THE OWNER COULD CATHETERIZE HIMSELF BY REMOVING THE FERRULE, THEN THE CATHETER FROM THE TIP. THE IVORY HANDLES HELD THE LUBRICANT. "PROSPECTIVES IN UROLOGY" VOL. I NOTES THAT THESE WERE PREPROSTATECTOMY DAYS AND SELF-CATHETERIZATION WAS NOT UNUSUAL. IT WAS MORE USUAL, HOWEVER, FOR THE CATHETER TO BE CARRIED IN THE SWEATBAND OF THE HAT. SALIVA LUBRICATED THE CATHETER BEFORE BEING USED.

THE CYSTOSCOPE

Two problems plagued the search for a workable cystoscope ~ casting enough light into the bladder's interior and the minute field of vision restricted by the narrow urethra. Philip Bozzini of Frankfort took up the challange in 1805 with his "Lichtleiter." His feeble candlelight did its best to illuminate the larynx (see "Laryngoscopes") through a hollow tube attachment. Another speculum, designed for introduction into the urinary tract, gave a very limited inspection of the female bladder and the male urethra.

TOP VIEW
REFLECTOR
CANDLE

1805
BOZZINI'S "LICHTLEITER"

SIDE VIEW
HOLDER HANDLE
REFLECTOR
SPECULUM
EYEPIECE
VERTICAL PARTITION
CANDLE HOLDER

(AMERICAN COLLEGE OF SURGEONS, CHICAGO)

The Bozzini "toy", as it was called, was roundly drubbed by the medical profession without realizing its potential.

M. Segalas revived the cystoscope concept before the Royal Academy of Sciences of France in 1826. Two small candles reflected light from a conical mirror into a polished urethral speculum. He told the assembled worthies that one could read the smallest printed type through the speculum at a distance of fifteen inches. Although considerably overstated, his enthusiasm was infectious. Perhaps the really workable cystoscope was just around the corner.

One year later, J.D. Fisher of Boston reflected candlelight from a perforated viewing mirror down a single tube. In 1853 Antonin Désormeaux embellished Fisher's concept with an alcohol and turpentine lamp. In addition, a concave mirror reflected this light through a planoconvex lens and into the eyepiece. There, a perforated viewing mirror reflected the rays down the urethral speculum. This endoscope was practical enough for the inventor to diagnose and treat urethritis, do an internal urethrotomy and remove a urethral papilloma. Although still advertized in Tiemann & Company's 1889 catalogue, it was mentioned that its considerable expense made it impractical for general use.

The preceeding endoscopes featured indirect vision~ that is, with the eye at an angle to the speculum axis, much like a periscope. In 1876, Max Nitze of Dresden produced the first functional direct vision cystoscope. His tube contained three channels with the center one providing direct viewing into the bladder. This and the upper channel carried circulating water to cool the heat from the lowest channel. It was the latter that held a lighting innovation~ a battery~supplied wire ending with a platinum loop ~ white-hot when the current was on. Glass windows at both ends of the cystoscope contained the water and permitted the brilliant light to illuminate the bladder. Adequate light ~ and where it was needed - was at last a reality.

1827

FISHER'S CYSTOSCOPE
(SHELLEY, PROSPECTIVES IN
UROLOGY, VOL. I 1976)

1853

DÉSORMEAUX'S CYSTOSCOPE
(SHELLEY, PROSPECTIVES IN
UROLOGY, VOL. I 1976)

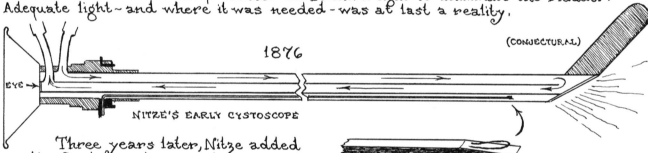

1876   (CONJECTURAL)

EYE →

NITZE'S EARLY CYSTOSCOPE

PLATINUM LOOP

Three years later, Nitze added the first true lens system as well as an interchangeable loop encased in a waterproof glass capsule. This was a real convenience because of frequent burnouts and fusing of the hot wire loop.

Nitze's third effort revived the old indirect viewing concept. A prism near the beak gave right-angle viewing. In the concave side of the beak itself was the platinum loop~ a position that gave that long sought larger field of vision. The circulating cooling water was, of course, still a necessity.

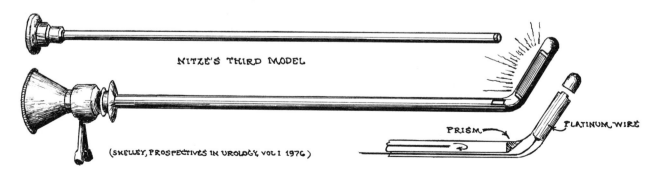

NITZE'S THIRD MODEL

PRISM   PLATINUM WIRE

(SHELLEY, PROSPECTIVES IN UROLOGY, VOL I 1976)

After Edison invented the incandescent bulb in 1880, David Newman of Glasgow was able to produce a bulb small enough to enter the bladder. His new direct vision design was a hollow vulcanite cone with a tip containing a glass lens. Once the bladder

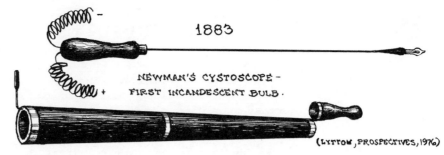

1883

NEWMAN'S CYSTOSCOPE - FIRST INCANDESCENT BULB.

(LYTTON, PROSPECTIVES, 1976)

was inspected, the tip could be pivoted out of the way with a rod that ran the length of the instrument. The bladder could then be treated or catheters passed into the ureters.

On this side of the Atlantic, cystoscopic imports seemed to satisfy the modest demand before the turn of the century. Less satisfying was the shipping of the instrument back to Europe for frequent repairs. Dr. William Otis pondered this inconvenience and a frequent trouble source~the Nitze right angle prism. It was practically impossible to make it permanently watertight. Otis proposed rounding the sides of the prism to give a wider angle of vision and better magnification. He impressed a New York instrument maker, Reinhold Wappler, with the idea. By 1900, America was producing its own version of the cystoscope. An added advantage was the very small wire passage to the bulb, thereby permitting a larger viewing lens system and a smaller overall diameter. New optical systems were subsequently developed for efficient forward and retrograde vision.

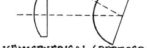

HEMISPHERICAL (RIGHT ANGLE)

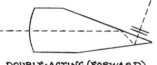

DOUBLE-ACTING (FORWARD)

HEMISPHERICAL (RETROGRADE)

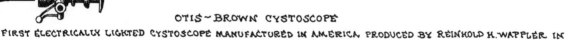

1900

REMOVABLE SHEATH

OTIS~BROWN CYSTOSCOPE

FIRST ELECTRICALLY LIGHTED CYSTOSCOPE MANUFACTURED IN AMERICA, PRODUCED BY REINHOLD H. WAPPLER IN COOPERATION WITH WILLIAM K. OTIS AND F. TILTON BROWN.

(AMERICAN CYSTOSCOPE MAKERS, INC. EQUIPMENT CATALOGUE 1952)

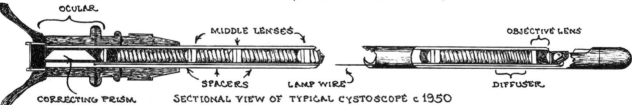

OCULAR.

MIDDLE LENSES

OBJECTIVE LENS

SPACERS   LAMP WIRE

DIFFUSER.

CORRECTING PRISM.   SECTIONAL VIEW OF TYPICAL CYSTOSCOPE c 1950

(AMERICAN CYSTOSCOPE MAKERS INC. CATALOGUE 1952)

The latest improvement came with the invention of the fiberotic bundle, first used in a cystoscope in the early 1960's. High optical glass fibers were coated with a lower density glass. Light entering each fiber struck the outer glass layer at less than a critical angle and therefore totally reflected down the fiber. A bundle of such fibers needed no fancy sets of prisms or lenses, and could be twisted without sacrificing the brilliant light or image reflection. Dr. Bozzini would have been most pleased to see his old external light source ideas working so efficiently with the new fiber optic concept!

THE SPIROMETER

Back in 1679, physiologist Borelli first experimented with the amount of air held in the lungs with a single deep inspiration. It proved a slow start in a long search to discover the air capacity of the normal expanded chest. Not until 1800 did Dr. Humphrey Davy measure his own residual volume (that air remaining in the lungs after maximum expiration) with his "Mercurial Air-Holding Machine."

The medical world finally took notice in 1846 when Dr. John Hutchinson published his On the Capacity of the Lungs and on Respiratory Function. Twenty years later, Austin Flint reviewed Hutchinson's investigations from an American viewpoint. In Flint's Physical Exploration of the Chest he stated that spirometry received its fullest development from Dr. Hutchinson.

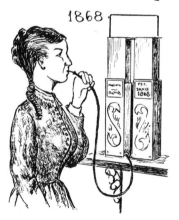

"It hinges on the fact that the lungs in health contain a certain volume of air which varies in a certain ratio with the height, age, and weight of the individual, and that anything which interferes with their permeability or their action will alter the volume of air they can be made to receive the exact amount of that interference.

MEASURING THE VITAL CAPACITY OF THE LUNGS
(JOHN HUTCHINSON'S ON THE CAPACITY OF THE LUNGS 1846)

The spirometer or instrument employed by Dr. Hutchinson for measuring what he terms the "vital capacity of the chest," or, in other words, the largest volume of air which the chest can be made to contain, consists of a cylinder closed at its upper extremity, and suspended in a reservoir of water by means of two cords fixed to opposite sides of the cylinder. Each cord passes over a pulley, and has a weight attached to its extremity; and the two weights are together sufficient to counterbalance the weight of the cylinder. When the instrument is ready for use, the cylinder is nearly but not quite full of water. A pipe, which forms a continuation of the tube through which the patient has to breathe, passes under the lower extremity of the cylinder, and rises within it above the level of the water. As the patient forces the air through this tube, each cubic inch of air which he expires displaces a corresponding amount of water, and raises the cylinder to a proportionate extent; and the exact amount of air discharged from the lungs in any given expiration is indicated by a graduated scale affixed."

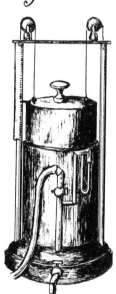

HUTCHINSON'S SPIROMETER
(TIEMANN & CO. 1889)

Dr. Flint went on to point out the pitfalls of assuming that a vital capacity outside the normal range actually indicated disease. Only if the patient had previous spirometry tests to compare with follow-up studies and not a general standard would the results be of real diagnostic value. Further, the vital capacity by itself gave no clues as to the nature of any lung disease. "Its indications are simply those of perfect or imperfect expansion of the lungs...."

BROWN'S SPIROMETER
(TIEMANN & CO 1889)

THERE ARE THREE TYPES OF SPIROMETERS ~
THE BELL WITH WATER BATH (PRECEEDING PAGE),
THE PISTON AND THE BELLOWS TYPES SHOWN HERE.

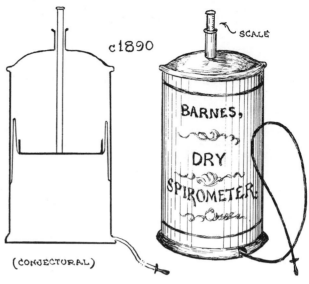

c1890

(CONJECTURAL)

PISTON TYPE OF SPIROMETER
(JOHN REYNDERS & CO. 1895)

Dr. Flint's evaluation of the spirometer's usefulness was on target for close to a century. Then the 1950's brought a fresh focus on lung volume measurement with the new electronics and computers. Newer gadgetry could relate the vital capacity to time. The healthy lung was found to empty in four seconds. 75% of this volume should be exhaled in the first second (FEV₁)

The troubled lung and its reduced vital capacity could then be classified as RESTRICTIVE and/or OBSTRUCTIVE disease. Restrictive problems (such as blood, pus and air in the pleural space, chest pain, lobectomy, phrenic nerve injury, and alveolar, interstitial or occlusive bronchial disease) prevented proper air intake. Exhaled air presented no difficulty. Therefore, if expired air were more than 75% the first second, restrictive disease was present.

On the other hand, obstructive lung disease (such as asthma, chronic obstructive disease, foreign bodies and bronchiectasis) with its characteristic wheeze, made exhaling difficult. It would be likely if less than 75% of the vital capacity were expired in one second. Bronchodilator medication could also be evaluated by recording pre and post-treatment measurements.

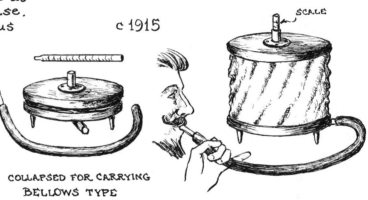

c 1915

COLLAPSED FOR CARRYING
BELLOWS TYPE
BOULITTE'S COMPACT SPIROMETER
(KNY-SCHEERER CO 1915)

c 1915 ~ 1950's

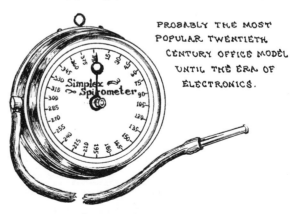

PROBABLY THE MOST POPULAR TWENTIETH CENTURY OFFICE MODEL UNTIL THE ERA OF ELECTRONICS.

SIMPLEX SPIROMETER
(KNY-SCHEERER CO. 1915)

1982

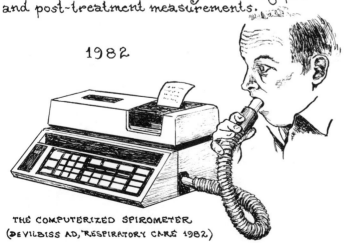

THE COMPUTERIZED SPIROMETER
(DEVILBISS AD, RESPIRATORY CARE 1982)

THERMOMETERS

It was clear to the ancients that bodily heat rose with illness and that a feverish patient was warm to the touch. Just HOW warm was a guesstimate. Some time between 1593~1597, Galileo thought up a simple apparatus that might actually measure one's temperature. When the patient's hand warmed an egg-sized glass bulb, the enclosed air expanded into the attached tube and bubbled out of a cup of water. On cooling, the water replaced the air to a level that varied with the heat of the hand. His "Thermoscope" unfortunately had barometer-like qualities, for the atmospheric pressure changes on the cup's water surface gave variable tube levels for the same patient. Still and all, Galileo had started the search for practical temperature measurements.

Santorio Santorio, concerned with the temperature fluctuations in health and disease, experimented with several ingenious devices to record the bodys heat by measuring not only that from the hand but also expired air and from the oral cavity. As Santorio said, the purpose was "···so that we can tell if the patient be better or worse."

c 1595

GALILEO'S
THERMOSCOPE.

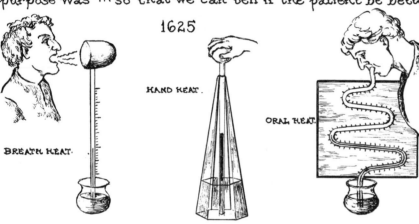

1625

BREATH HEAT.

HAND HEAT.

ORAL HEAT.

SANTORIO'S THERMOMETERS (AFTER REISER, MEDICINE AND THE REIGN OF TECHNOLOGY 1978)

By the mid 1600's, the fluid column had been completely sealed in the bulb and tube. Atmospheric pressure was no longer a consideration. But there were other head-scratchers, the most immediate being to decide on the most responsive fluid to use as well as choosing temperature constants upon which a degree scale could be based.

THE LIQUID ~ Wine spirits proved unsatisfactory, for this liquid froze quickly and boiled at a low temperature. Linseed oil was also a second best, for it smeared the glass tube bore. The clear preference was mercury ~ it never froze, boiled only with extreme heat, did not coat the bore and reacted promptly to cold and heat.

THE SCALE ~ In 1708 Dutch inventor, Gabriel Fahrenheit chose three fixed points for his temperature scale. A mixture of ice and sea water gave zero degrees, the freezing point of water was 32 degrees, and the normal body temperature at 96.6 degrees (initially 90, then 96 degrees had been chosen). Because the boiling temperature at 212 degrees varied with the atmospheric pressure, it was ruled out as a reliable constant. For convenience sake, the scale was divided into 96 equal parts. The Fahrenheit scale proved reliable when a patient's temperature was identical with several of his calibrated instruments.

1X   PAPER SCALE

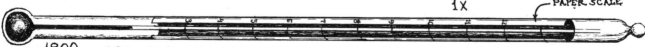

c 1800 TYPE DEVISED BY JOHN HUNTER FOR ANIMAL OBSERVATIONS. FAHRENHEIT SCALE.
(WELLCOME MUSEUM, LONDON)

─ IVORY SCALE OUTSIDE GLASS TUBE.

1X

c1800 UNDERARM THERMOMETER OF THE TYPE USED BY JAMES CURRIE IN HIS COLD
WATER TREATMENT OF FEVERS. FAHRENHEIT SCALE. (WELLCOME MUSEUM, LONDON).

There were other possibilities, and in 1742 Swedish scientist Celsius chose
zero for boiling water and 100 degrees for the freezing point of water. In
this way, the scale divided nicely into 100 degree markings. Shortly after
the scale was reversed, although still known as the Celsius scale. Comparing
this to the Fahrenheit thermometer, the normal body temperature was 37 degrees
centigrade or 98.6 degrees F.

$\frac{7}{8}$X

Thermometer fur Franken Diagnose nach Celsius

c1780 THERMOMETER BELONGING TO WILLIAM CULLEN, M.D., USED IN WARDS IN HIS HOSPITAL
BEFORE INTRODUCTION OF CLINICAL THERMOMETRY AS A SYSTEM. CELSIUS SCALE. (MUTTER MUSEUM, PHILADELPHIA).

The average practicing physician digested these efforts and felt the thermometer was too clumsy (some were a foot long), inaccurate (there was no universal
testing standard for the accuracy of the individual instrument) and time-consuming
(many took twenty minutes to register).

Another target for this not unfounded criticism was the bent thermometer of
the eighteenth and early nineteenth century. Designed to take the axillary (armpit)
temperature, its scale on an ivory or bone strip could be read only if in place. If
removed before recording, the mercury column might well drop in the process and
give a false reading. The lengthy oral thermometer suffered the same flaw unless
the physician bent his back for an on-site recording.

SELF-REGISTERING OR INDEX THERMOMETER. ~ Geology professor John Phillips of
Oxford added to the considerable efforts of German and other European investigators after twenty years of experimentation. In 1851 he presented his self-registering or index thermometer at the Great Exhibition. The index referred to a bit of mercury
that was separated from the main column by a tiny air bubble. When pushed up
by the expanded column, it remained in position to indicate the degree of temperature. Phillips' idea moldered until about 1850, when William Aitkin of the Royal
Victoria Hospital had a self-registering thermometer made for clinical trial.
It was outsized ~ a full ten inches long ~ on the thought that with a wider
degree scale, the index would be less likely to be shaken down into the bulb.

For the remainder of the century, English innovations and accuracy
were highly prized on both sides of the Atlantic. This was the state of
affairs when the Civil War tore the United States ~ and countless of its young
men ~ apart. Although the thermometer's potential had yet to be realized, a Dr.
Billings first used a ten inch instrument at the Seven Days Battle near Richmond.
There is no account as to how the doctor was able to carry the lengthy glass stick
safely from battlefield to battlefield. Perhaps it was boxed as shown here.

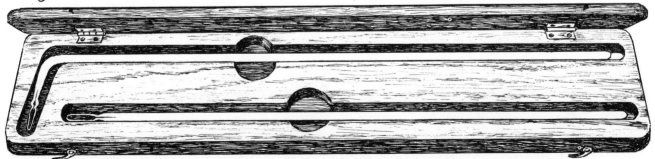

1865 THERMOMETERS OF THE TYPE USED BY WILLIAM AITKIN. (WELLCOME MUSEUM, LONDON).

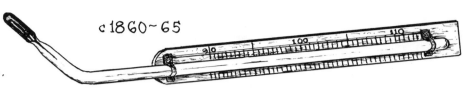

CLINICAL THERMOMETER OF
THE CIVIL WAR PERIOD. THE
SCALE IS ATTACHED AND NOT
ETCHED INTO THE GLASS. AXILLA.
(MUTTER MUSEUM, PHILADELPHIA.)

c 1860~65

SIZE ~ Big certainly wasn't best, and practicing physician Sir Thomas Allbutt proved it in 1867. He had a "short" six inch thermometer made that could register the index in five minutes. Soon after he produced a three inch instrument-the prototype of today's clinical thermometers. Within a decade, the number of imports had jumped from fifty to over three thousand a year. A small, fast, accurate, self-recording thermometer had reached the American market~ a practical addition for any practice.

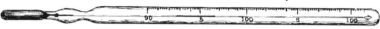

c 1870 ALLBUTT THERMOMETER.

(ASHHURST, INTERNATIONAL ENCYCLOPAEDIA OF SURGERY VOL. I 1881)

READABILITY ~ A problem remained, however, for the fine column of mercury that now reacted so quickly to bodily heat was difficult to read. About 1877, Hicks of London laid in a prismatic glass strip that could magnify the index to 100X. The modern thermometer had arrived.

c 1880 HICKS' SELF-REGISTERING
INDESTRUCTIBLE INDEX THERMOMETER.

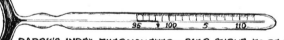

(SHARP & SMITH, CHICAGO 1889)

Old predjudices had to be countered if its potential was to be realized. A young Leipzig physician, Carl Wunderlich, championed the cause early on by taking regular temperature readings of his hospital patients. He wrote of his findings in his 1868 classic which was translated into English in 1871 and entitled "On the Temperature in Diseases." His scientific analysis of the body's temperature in health and diseases convinced many that this important diagnostic tool should rank with the microscope and the stethoscope.

CERTIFICATION ~ As the number of thermometer makers increased in response to the demand, the accuracy came into question. Physicians needed some sort of quality guarantee and American manufacturers were in want of certification if they were to compete with the English. In 1880, the Thermometric Bureau of Yale College of New Haven began the certification and issued a certificate of accuracy for each instrument that met its standards. With such a guarantee, physicians had little need to import thermometers.

Here are some unusual thermometers offered before the turn of the century.

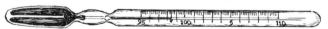

SEGUIN'S SURFACE THERMOMETER, SELF-REGISTERING
ZERO AT NORMAL TEMPERATURE. (TIEMANN & CO. 1889)

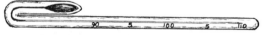

BENT THERMOMETER. (TIEMANN & CO. 1889)

DOUBLE BULB ~ GAVE EXTRA SURFACE EXPOSURE FOR MORE
RAPID MERCURY EXPANSION. THE LARGE BORE MADE INDEX
READING EASIER. (SHARP & SMITH, CHICAGO 1889)

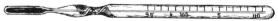

PATENT TWIST STEM THERMOMETER. (TIEMANN & CO. 1889)

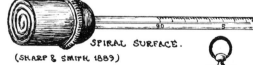

BARRY'S INDEX THERMOMETER ~ BULB CURVE TO REST
UNDER THE TONGUE AND DISTRIBUTE HEAT EVENLY.
(REYNDERS & CO. 1895)

SPIRAL SURFACE.

(SHARP & SMITH 1889)

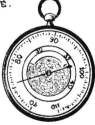

IMMISCH'S AVITREOUS SURFACE
THERMOMETER FOR MOUTH OR AXILLA.
EXPANSIVE LIQUIDS ARE IN A METAL
TUBE THAT EXPANDS WITH HEAT.
(SHARP & SMITH 1889)

THE DOCTOR'S BAG

Diagnostic instruments were late bloomers on the medical scene. They were few enough in the nineteenth century to be carried in the hat or pocket, as in the case of the stethoscope. But when the early twentieth century physician set out on house calls, there weren't enough pockets to hold his hetero-geneous collection of reflex hammers, sphygmomanometer, ophthalmoscope, tonometer, otoscope, nasal speculum, head mirror, tongue depressors, various specula and perhaps an endoscope, as well as a thermometer or two and assorted medicines. It was then that the doctor's bag came into it's own.

The history of containers for surgical instruments and medicines date back to much earlier days. Our American Indian shamans filled their medicine bags with an unusual assortment of curative objects. From excavated Pompeii and other ruins came evidence of scalpels packed head to tail in wooden boxes. There were probes, forceps, spatulas, hooks, sounds and forceps in cylindrical bronze cases, and medicines in pocket-sized rectangular bronze boxes.

The demand for surgeons exploded in the fifteenth century with the invention of gunpowder. They brought their skills to the destruction on the battlefield ~ and large portable chests to hold their instruments. Smaller cases ~ "plaister boxes" ~ were more easily carried by seventeenth century surgeons. The upper and larger compartment accommodated the variety of instruments, while the lower held salves and wads of cloth fibers or lint for dressings.

EARLY AMERICAN CHESTS, both surgical and medical, saw considerable service in the American Revolution. These ranged from plain make-do boxes, some up to three feet long, to finely crafted hardwood chest with brass furniture. Some were faced with leather.

1830
BLACKFOOT INDIAN
MEDICINE MAN WITH
ANIMAL MEDICINE BAG.
(AFTER GEORGE CATLIN)

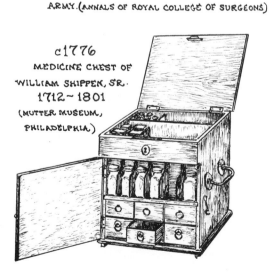

c1570

CHEST USED BY WILLIAM CLOWES (1544-1604)
WHILE SURGEON IN EARL OF WARWICK'S
ARMY. (ANNALS OF ROYAL COLLEGE OF SURGEONS)

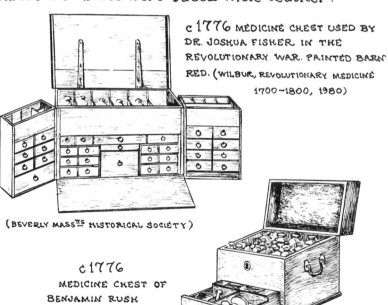

c1776 MEDICINE CHEST USED BY
DR. JOSHUA FISHER IN THE
REVOLUTIONARY WAR. PAINTED BARN
RED. (WILBUR, REVOLUTIONARY MEDICINE
1700~1800, 1980)

(BEVERLY MASS^TS HISTORICAL SOCIETY)

c1776
MEDICINE CHEST OF
BENJAMIN RUSH
(MUTTER MUSEUM, PHILADELPHIA)

c1776
MEDICINE CHEST OF
WILLIAM SHIPPEN, SR.
1712~1801
(MUTTER MUSEUM,
PHILADELPHIA)

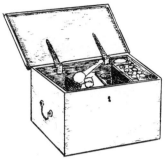

AMERICAN HALF CHEST OF THE
TYPE USED IN THE REVOLUTION.
(WEST POINT MUSEUM, NEW YORK.)

L 12", H 6", W 8"

Smaller field chests of the Revolution were 10-12 inches square and 8-10 inches in height. Some were partitioned with holes for medicine vials, and there were those with drawers for minor surgical instruments, a set of weights and scales, and a pill roller square of tile or glass. Many chests were sold by colonial apothecaries completely outfitted with medicines.

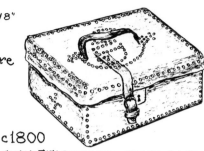

c 1800

SMALL FIELD MEDICAL CHEST — WOOD
AND LEATHER COVERED WITH M.D.
DESIGN IN BRASS TACKS.
(DR. WILLIAM BEAUMONT HOMESTEAD, LEBANON, CONN II)

NINETEENTH CENTURY CHESTS ~
Homeopathy was brought to New York City in 1825 by Dr. Hans Burch Gram. Some medicines, when used in excess, produced similar symptoms to those of a particular illness. Homeopathy held that minute amounts of those medicines that matched the symptoms should be given. In a day when underlying pathology was unknown, symptomatic treatment was

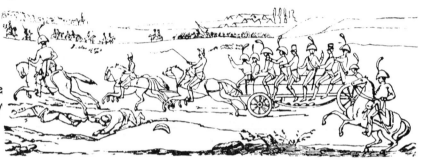

NAPOLEON'S ARMY PHYSICIANS RODE INTO BATTLE ON THEIR MOBILE MEDICAL CHEST.
(BETTMANN, PICTORIAL HISTORY OF MEDICINE 1956)

appealing. A large chest that would accommodate the hundreds of vials was a necessity. Until medical diagnosis became more precise, many such chests were used in the Civil War.

Homeopathic medicine chests were also sold for home use well into the twentieth century. Each vial was usually labeled with the name of the drug and a number. A book was included so that the patient could match his symptoms with the numbered vials for a sort of cookbook therapy.

c 1860

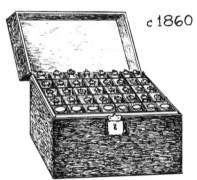

CIVIL WAR FIELD CHEST.

c 1900

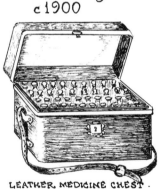

LEATHER MEDICINE CHEST.
(LENTZ & CO. SONS, PHILADELPHIA)

c 1910

10" X 6" X 8"

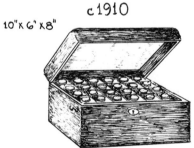

HOUSEHOLD HOMEOPATHIC CHEST
SOLD BY WHITEALL TATUM.
(RICHARDSON, PILL ROLLERS, 1979)

CASES ~ In the eighteenth and nineteenth centuries, surgical sets were carried in elongated oblong wooden boxes with lid handles. The homeopathic emphasis in the early 1800's also produced multi-vialed cases, then replaced by smaller containers as specific disease therapy became known.

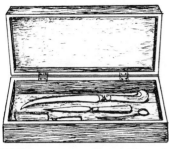

1777 MILITARY SURGEON'S CASE
OF PETER TURNER, M.D., 1ST R.I.
REGIMENT AND CHARLES GREEN, M.D.,
HOSPITAL DEPARTMENT (HISTORICAL
MUSEUM OF MEDICINE + DENTISTRY, HARTFORD)

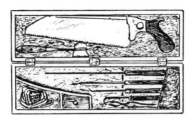

c1860 CIVIL WAR SURGICAL
CASE (DAMMANN, CIVIL WAR
INSTRUMENTS& EQUIPMENT, 1983)

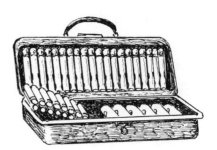

1917 LEATHER MEDICINE CASE
L 17" x H 6" x W 5½"
(BECTON, DICKINSON & CO, RUTHERFORD, N.J.)

SMALL POCKET CASES ~ The following were easily
carried into battle or on emergency calls.

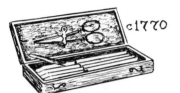

CASE OF SCISSORS AND
SCALPELS (ARMED FORCES
INSTITUTE OF PATHOLOGY)

c1770

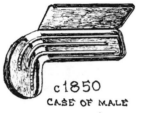

c1850
CASE OF MALE
CATHETERS (HISTORICAL
MUSEUM OF MEDICINE & DENTISTRY, HARTFORD)

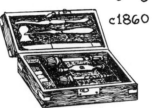

c1860

TREPANNING SET, CIVIL
WAR ~ DR. VILES.
(AUTHORS)

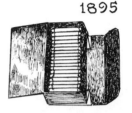

1895

POCKET MEDICINE CASE,
LEATHER 8⅛" x 3⅝" x 1⅛"
(REYNDERS & CO. 1895)

WALLETS ~ These soft pocket cases carried medicines and instruments conveniently.
Wales, in his 1867 Mechanical Therapeutics, described a typical surgical wallet
used by Naval medical officers on Civil War expeditions. The wallet was a piece of
strong leather three feet long and fourteen inches wide. When rolled, a strap
could be hooked to both ends and slung over the shoulder or hand-carried. It held
two pint flasks with screw tops, one for chloroform and the other, brandy. There was
also a half pint flask of aqua ammonia, amputation knife, a small saw, bone
forceps, three screw and six field tourniquets, twelve roller bandages, four yards
of muslin, one lot of maltese crosses and other compresses, six yards of
adhesive plaster, twelve short splints and one box of simple cerate.

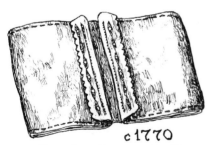

c1770
LEATHER MEDICAL WALLET.
WASHINGTON'S HEADQUARTERS, NEWBURGH, N.Y.
(WILBUR, CONTINENTAL SOLDIER 1969)

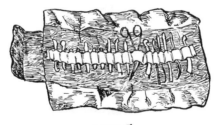

1825
SURGICAL POCKET CASE.
(MUSEUM OF MEDICINE & SURGERY, CONN.)

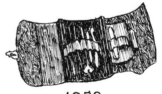

1850
SURGICAL POCKET CASE.
(HISTORICAL MUSEUM OF MEDICINE +
DENTISTRY, HARTFORD, CONN.)

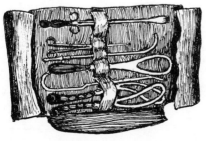

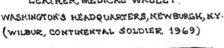

c1855
OBSTETRICAL
POUCH.
(MUSEUM OF MEDICINE
+ DENTISTRY, CONN.)

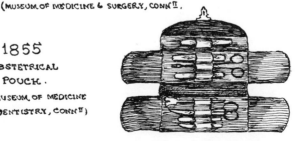

c1860
CIVIL WAR CASE.
(AUTHOR)

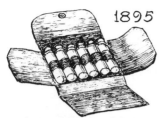

1895

POCKET MEDICINE CASE.
CLOSURE SNAPS REPLACED
CLASPS BY 1875~80
(REYNDERS & CO. 1895)

1900

LEATHER COVERED HARD CASE.
SMALL POCKET SIZES TO LARGER FOR
BUGGY BAGS   (PARK DAVIS CO. 1900)

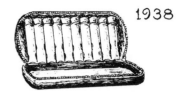

1938

LEATHER CASED VIALS FOR
PHYSICIAN'S BAG. NOTE ZIPPER
CLOSURE, NEW IN THE 1930'S.
(MUELLER & CO. 1938)

BAGS ~ To my knowledge, the earliest American medical bag was that of Dr. David Townsend's (1753-1839). Although in the Massachusetts Medical Library of Boston for many years, its whereabouts is unknown to me. Twelve inches deep and six inches across, it was of human skin from a pirate hanged on Boston Common. It was a grim reminder of the days when little sympathy was spent on high sea outlaws, and the old Yankee saying "waste not, want not."

Medical and surgical saddle bags were particularly useful for the physician on horseback. Draped over the animal's neck, the rider could make his horse-or rather house-calls with all manner of instruments and medicines to meet the back country emergencies.

1517

SURGEON'S ASSISTANT PACKING
DOCTOR'S BAG WITH SALVES AND
POWDERS. AFTER GERSDORFF 1517.
(BETTMANN, PICTORIAL HISTORY OF MEDICINE 1956)

1800

SADDLE BAG USED BY
DR. ELEZEAR POMEROY
HUNT, WHO PRACTICED
IN TOLLAND COUNTY,
CONN̄ FOR 67 YEARS.
(HISTORICAL MUSEUM OF
MEDICINE AND
DENTISTRY, CONN̄)

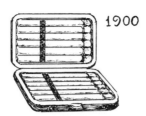

Chunky homeopathic bags were probably in use in the 1840's. Better diagnostic instruments gradually made medical shotgun therapy obsolete, and with it the multi-vialed bag by the 1880's. Replacing it were satchel-like bags, carrying many of the diagnostic tools of medicine familiar today.

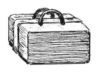

c 1840-1880
HOMEOPATHIC

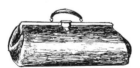

c 1880~1930±
OBSTETRICAL

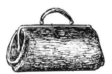

c 1880~1940±
ENGLISH STYLE

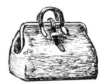

c 1880~1984+
BOSTON

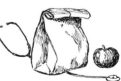

c 1900~1945±
CLUB STYLE

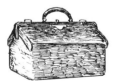

c 1880~1930
CABIN STYLE

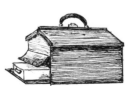

c 1925~1945
COMBINATION
WITH COPPER STERILIZER

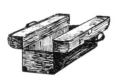

c 1930~1950±
PANDORA
COMPARTMENTED BAG

c 1930-1970±
UTILITY KIT

c 1975~1984+
PLEASE REFRIGERATE
(WORCESTER MEDICAL LIBRARY)

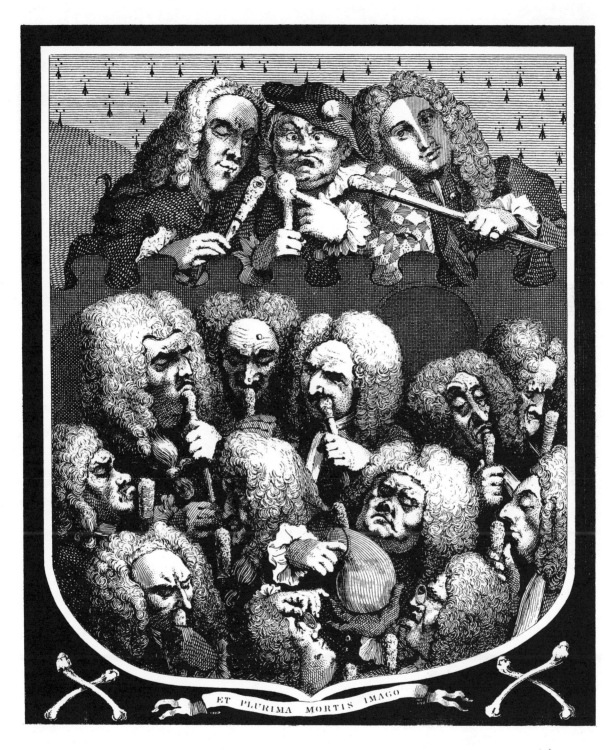

ET PLURIMA MORTIS IMAGO

Hogarth's "Consultation of Physicians" seem to have a weighty diagnosis near at hand. The learned assembly will next turn to their

THERAPEUTIC MEDICAL INSTRUMENTS.

FORCEPS

AN INSTRUMENT FOR SEIZING AND MAKING COMPRESSION OR TRACTION, FROM THE LATIN — CIPIS, DERIVED FROM FERRUM (IRON) OR FORMUS (HOT) AND CAPIO (I TAKE), THEREFORE AN IRON FOR SEIZING OR SEIZING SOMETHING HOT.

Some unheralded prehistoric cook probably found that hot coals could be plucked from the fire with a green bent stick. These make shift tongs had the grasping function of the thumb and forefinger without burning or blistering. The Egyptians at least five thousand years ago were using a bent strip of iron or bronze for epilation. Its surgical implications were not lost in later years.

DRESSING, TISSUE AND SPLINTER FORCEPS

Dressing forceps are not only used for dressing wounds but also for removing injured tissue and small foreign bodies. The earliest was the thumb forceps, otherwise known as tweezers, simple or spring forceps. The axis hinge, like that of the scissors, was a later dressing forceps innovation.

As needs became more specialized, the tips of the blades determined the function. Dressing forceps had grooved inner surfaces, tissue forceps were toothed for better grasping, and splinter forceps had inner grooves on finely-pointed ends.

DRESSING FORCEPS.   TISSUE (MOUSE-TOOTHED).   SPLINTER FORCEPS.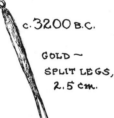

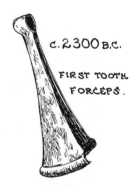

c. 3300 B.C.

BRONZE & COPPER SPRING LOOP.

EGYPTIAN.
(McFADDEN, ··· SPRING FORCEPS 1970)

c. 3200 B.C.

GOLD ~
SPLIT LEGS,
2.5 CM.

DYNASTY OF UR,
MESOPOTAMIA.
(McFADDEN, ··· SPRING FORCEPS, 1970)

c. 2750 B.C.

2 BRONZE STRIPS
FASTENED AT TOP.
7 CM. LONG.

LOST CITY OF BISMAYAH,
MESOPOTAMIA,
(McFADDEN, ··· SPRING FORCEPS, 1970)

c. 2300 B.C.

FIRST TOOTH
FORCEPS.

TOMB OF MESARA,
CRETE.
(McFADDEN, ··· FORCEPS, 1970)

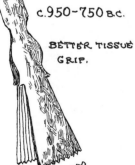

c. 950-750 B.C.

BETTER TISSUE
GRIP.

BRONZE AGE, LÜNEBURG,
GERMANY.
(McFADDEN, ··· FORCEPS, 1970)

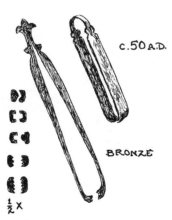

½ X

c. 50 A.D.

BRONZE

ROMAN TOOTH FORCEPS -
EVOLVED FROM CRETAN.
(McFADDEN, ··· FORCEPS 1970)

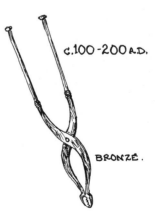

c. 100-200 A.D.

BRONZE.

ROMAN ~ FROM POMPEII.
(THOMPSON - HISTORY OF
SURGICAL INSTRUMENTS, 1941)

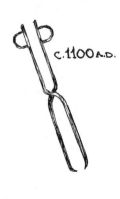

c. 1100 A.D.

FORCEPS FROM A
MANUSCRIPT - ALBUCASIS.
(THOMPSON - HISTORY OF
SURGICAL INSTRUMENTS,
1941)

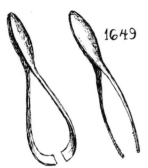

1649

DRESSING   TISSUE
(JOSEPH SCHMID – INSTRUMENTA
CHIRURGICA, AUGSBURG 1649)

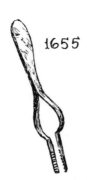

1655

FOREIGN BODY FORCEPS WITH
HANDLE SPATULA FOR SPREADING
OINTMENT OR PLASTER ON LINEN
(SCULTETUS, ARMAMENTARIUM 1655)

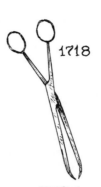

1718

TISSUE
LORENZ HEISTER
(CHIRURGIE, NÜRNBURG 1718)

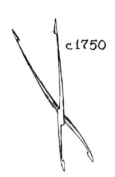

c 1750

DOUBLE-ENDED TISSUE
(BENNION-ANTIQUE MED.
INSTRUMENTS 1979)

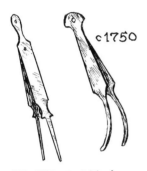

c1750

SPLINTER-DRESSING
DR. CHRISTOPHER HEYDRICK'S,
PHILADELPHIA
(MUTTER MUSEUM, PHILADELPHIA)

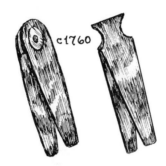

c1760

DRESSING – TORTOISE SHELL
(FORT TICONDEROGA MUSEUM,
TICONDEROGA, N.Y.)

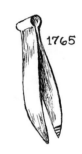

c 1760~70

REVOLUTIONARY WAR
(ARMED FORCES INS. PATHOLOGY)

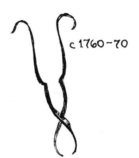

1765

DRESSING
(DIDEROT'S
ENCYCLOPEDIA 1765)

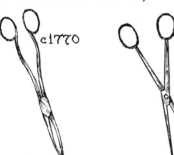

c1770

DR. CHRISTOPHER HEYDRICK'S
(MUTTER MUSEUM, PHILADELPHIA)

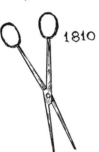

1810

"COMMON FORCEPS"
(LONGMAN, HURST, REES,
& ORME, LONDON 1810)

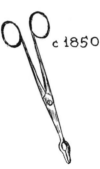

c 1850

POLYPUS FORCEPS
FOR NASAL POLYPS.
(SMITH – PRINCIPLES-PRACTICE OF SURGERY, PHIL. 1863)

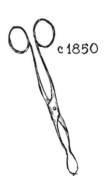

c 1850

TUMOR FORCEPS

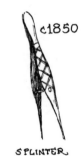

c1850

SPLINTER
(DUNGLISON – DICTIONARY
OF MED. SCIENCE, PHIL 1854)

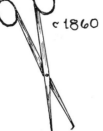

c. 1860

DRESSING
(WALES – SURGERY, 1867)

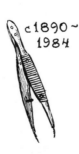

c 1860

HOOK SPLINTER FORCEPS
(ERUCHSEN – SURGERY 1869)

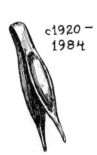

c 1890~
1984

SPLINTER
(REYNDER + CO, N.Y. 1895)

c 1920~
1984

FEILCHENFELD'S SPLINTER
(REID BROS 1925)

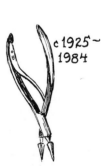

c 1925~
1984

"VIRTUS" SPLINTER
(MUELLER CO 1938)

89

ARTERY FORCEPS

William Steward Halsted wrote in the 1912 "Bulletin of the Johns Hopkins Hospital" that "The only weapon with which the unconcious patient can immediately retaliate upon the incompetent surgeon is hemorrhage." When fumbling fingers were added to the early methods to stem those bloody gushers, the result must have been devastating.

It is true that ligatures were occasionally used by the Romans, but thereafter the technique was generally ignored in favor of cauderization (also used by the Greeks and Romans). Without benefit of anesthesia, the bleeder was cooked with a red-hot iron. The artery and adjacent tissues were blocked by a thick slough or eschar, which

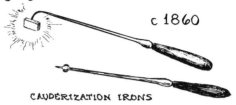

c 1860

CAUDERIZATION IRONS

might well bleed again in six to eight days when the slough separated. Hot knives, boiling pitch, oil and molten lead were also accepted methods for hemostasis.

Ambroise Paré, when he became a French military surgeon in 1536, rebelled against such barbarism on the battlefield. He later wrote in his <u>The Apologie and Treatise of Ambroise Paré</u> "...that one cannot apply hot irons but with extreame and vehement pains in a sensible part, void of a Gangreene which would be cause of a Convulsion, Feaver, yea, oft times of death." He recalled the scattered use of ligatures by ancient worthies, used the technique in his surgery and then wrote of his considerable successes. Paré included this illustration of his own invention with the caption "The Crowes beake fit for to draw the vessells forth of the flesh wherein they lye hid, that they may be tyed or bound fast."

1585
"CROWES BEAKE"

Paré had made a strong case for the use of ligatures, but acceptance was painfully slow. Sharp, writing in his 1761 "A Critical Enquiry into the Present State of Surgery" was distressed to find that ligation instead of caudery "...was not universally practiced amongst surgeons residing in the more distant counties of our kingdom." The lack of enthusiasm frequently followed failure from not tying the ligature tightly due to the fear that the coats of the artery would be injured and weakened.

1607~1700
CROW'S BEAK WITH SPRING,
EXCAVATED AT JAMESTOWN
(NATIONAL PARK SERVICE)

Caudery still saw service during the American Civil War although a rarity. Only if soft and porous tissue were hemorrhaging and would not hold a ligature, or if many small vessels were bleeding at the same time would caudery be considered.

The growing number of surgeons who appreciated Paré's recommendations preferred the tenaculum. The hook-like instrument was used to seize the bleeding vessel and pull it outward for tying. Unfortunately, groping for the retracted vessel sometimes resulted in several puntures that could later ulcerate and hemorrhage. What was needed was a forceps that would function as Paré's "crowes beake" but was small, self-closing and applied with one hand.

1884

A LATER TENACULUM
(BRYANT-OPERATIVE
SURGERY 1884)

Three locking possibilities had surfaced by the early 1800's:

ROMAN

BOTH
c 800~400 BC.
SLIDING-RING LOCKS
(McFADDEN - ORIGIN+EVOLUTION-SPRING FORCEPS 1970)

1655
SCREW FORCEPS
(SCULTETUS-ARMAMENTARIUM 1655)

BENJAMIN BELL'S

1807
SLIDING SLOT FORCEPS
(THOMPSON- HIST. SURG. INST. 1941)

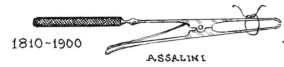

1810~1900

ASSALINI

About 1830, Joseph Frederic Charrière invented the first practical locking forceps. When an artery was clamped, a knobbed spring locked both arms securely in a closed position. It was innovative and efficient, and shortly after, Fricke produced forceps with a slide catch for locking. Langenbeck's version used a sliding pin catch.

1830~1900   SPRING CATCH.

c1835~1915   SLIDE CATCH.

c1835~1915   PINION CATCH.

CHARRIÈRE'S   FRICKE'S   LANGENBECK'S
(ALL FROM FOSTER MEDICAL DICTIONARY 1891)

The wave of arterial forceps crested in 1840 with Charrière's crossed leg forceps. Here was an entirely new design that was non-crushing, self-closing, self-holding and easily applied with one hand. Dieffenbach, a Berlin physician, introduced his broad-legged version in 1845. And that same year, Liston used Charrière's spring catch with toothed ends to secure bleeders on a flat surface.

1840~1900   1845~1915   1845

LISTON'S SECURED BLEEDING POINTS ON A FLAT SURFACE.

c1850~1915

CHARRIÈRE FORCEPS WITH CROSSED LEGS.
(McFADDEN...SPRING FORCEPS 1970)

DIEFFENBACH'S ARTERY FORCEPS
(McFADDEN...SPRING FORCEPS 1970)

LISTON'S "BULLDOG* FORCEPS
(WELLCOME MUSEUM, LONDON)

LISTON'S LATER MODEL
(BRYANT...SURGERY 1883)

*"BULLDOG" IS A LOOSE TERM FOR FORCEPS WITH JAWS AT THE LEGS' ENDS FOR GRASPING AND THEREFORE APPLIES TO ANY TOOTHED SELF-RETAINING FORCEPS, ESPECIALLY THE EARLIER LISTON AND DIEFFENBACH MODELS. IN AMERICA TODAY, "BULLDOG" MEANS ANY SELF-CLOSING, SELF-HOLDING, CROSSED OR UNCROSSED LEGS WITH BULLDOG-LIKE TEETH OR SERRATIONS.

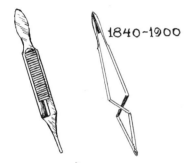

1848

CASSIS

2 PATTERNS OF SERRÉFINES
(PYE-SURGICAL HANDICRAFT, VOL. 1892)

In 1848, two different types of clips or serréfines proved helpful for the quick clamping of a bleeder. These were small enough to leave on the small arteries until all bleeding ceased, or the surgeon could return at his convenience to tie any vessels that might later bleed.

Until the middle of the nineteenth century, the tenaculum had been in general use. As late as 1873, Lister noted that this arterial hook was still in limited service, although largely replaced by Robert Liston's catch forceps ~ but it took some forty years after its introduction.

Immediately popular was Liston's 1850 fenestrated forceps. A ligature could be handily slipped over a clamped artery that was deeply seated such as between bones. The pouch of tissue that bulged through the fenestration prevented a loss of grip.

c1850~1915

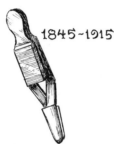

LISTON'S FENESTRATED "BULLDOG"
(ERICHSEN, SCIENCE, ART OF SURGERY 1854)

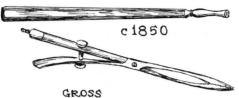

c1850

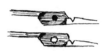

c1850~1930

GROSS

AFTER ATTACHING TO A BLEEDING POINT,
THE HANDLE WAS UNSCREWED AND THE BLADES
LEFT IN PLACE UNTIL ALL DANGER OF
BLEEDING WAS OVER.
(BRYANT - OPERATIVE SURGERY 1884)

France's Dr. Pean bucked the
strong arterial spring forceps
trend in the mid nineteenth
century with his axis hinged
instruments. It differed from
those with scissor arms of the
previous century in that the
forceps could be locked in
the closed position. The
narrow grooved blades made for
a sure hold on the artery.

PEAN'S
(WELLCOME MUSEUM, LONDON)

There was no need for Pean's pre-
sterilization era forceps to be disassembed, for
bacterial contamination was unknown at that time. Later so-called hemostatic or
pressure forceps had break-apart joints for easier cleaning and sterilization.

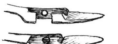

PIVOT SCREW OR RIVET.
BEFORE 1880

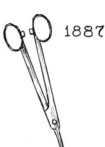

HEMISPHERIC JOINT.
c1880~1900

BOX JOINT.
c1860~1900

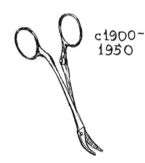

ASEPTIC JOINT.
c1900~1950

With better sterilization methods, the pivot screw staged a comeback around 1890.

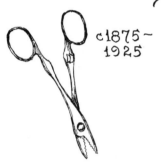

c1875~ 1925

LAWSON TAIT
WITH BOX JOINT.

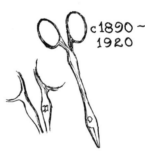

1887

SIR SPENCER-WELLS
SHORT-TOOTHED BLADES.

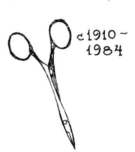

c1890~ 1920

SPENCER-WELLS
IMPROVED LOCK.

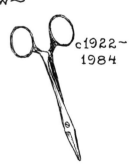

c1900~ 1950

SPENCER-WELLS
CURVED BLADES-ASEPTIC JOINT.

(THOMPSON - HISTORY OF SURGICAL INSTRUMENTS 1941)

The popular Spencer-Wells arterial forceps could also double as sponge
or needle-holding forceps.

A few more recent and more familiar arterial forceps follow~

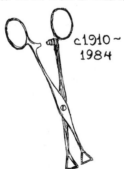

c1910~ 1984

**HALSTEAD ~ WITH
EARLIER BOX JOINT.**
(KNY-SCHEERER CO. 1915)

c1910~ 1984

PENNINGTON'S
(KNY-SCHEERER CO. 1915)

c1910~ 1984

HALSTEAD'S MOSQUITO
(REID BROS. 1915)

c1922~ 1984

KELLY
(SHARP AND SMITH 1925)

NEEDLE HOLDERS

In earlier days, these instruments served to grasp a needle for suturing any deep area of the body not easily reached for tying ligatures with the fingers. Such forceps were rare indeed before Joseph Lister's monumental development of surgical antiseptics in 1865. Indeed, the patient unfortunate enough to undergo internal surgery with a germ-laden scalpel courted sepsis and death.

Even as late as 1874, a leading British surgeon spoke of "those portions of the human frame that will ever be sacred." He went on to say that "...the abdomen, the chest and the brain would be for- ever shut from the intrusion of the wise and humane surgeon." The survival odds were dismal, two to one against recovery. Needle holders, therefore, remained low on one's instrument priority list!

CHIRURGIE, PLATE III
(DIDEROT'S ENCYCLOPEDIA 1765)

Yet there were those pioneering spirits who placed necessity before statistics. America's Ephraim McDowell, for example, performed the first ovariotomy in 1809. Although he did not describe his instruments, it is possible that he had in hand one of the new Physick needle holders.

EARLY 1800's

Philip Syng Physick was John Hunter's favorite American pupil. In 1792 he returned from London and Edinburgh to Philadelphia fairly bursting with surgical innovations. He was one of the first to wash out a stomach, using a long flexible tube and pewter syringe. He devised a wire snare for removing tonsils, a splint for fractured thighs and another for elbows, and a cannula for drawing off excess fluids from the brain through a trephine hole in the skull.

In 1816, Dr. Physick reintroduced Galen's old catgut sutures to replace the use of deep, non-absorbable silk or linen thread then in fashion. The catgut and his needle "carriers" saw considerable service in tying off large arteries. Dr. Nathan Smith, in his Memoirs of 1831, recalled the ligation of the external iliac artery. "By means of Dr. Physick's curved forceps, I then passed the aneurism under the artery...." The instrument lacked only a better locking device to make it practical today.

PHYSICK'S FORCEPS AND NEEDLE.
(SMITH, "PRACTICE OF SURGERY, 1863)

Anesthesia, Lister's anti- septic techniques, Robert Koch's proof that bacteria could indeed be the cause for infection all were advances paving the way for a complete surgical revolution. Needle holders became a must for careful and calculated internal surgery and for twenty years everything but pliers seemed to be considered as a possible needle-gripping instrument. Most were of the scissors axis pivot type much like the Spencer-Wells arterial forceps of 1887, but with a variety of locking devices and jaws for clamping.

c 1880   c 1880   c 1880

SNAP LOCK.

POST-LISTER NEEDLE FORCEPS OR HOLDERS.
(BRYANT, MANUAL OF OPERATIVE SURGERY VOL I, 1884)

These needle forceps worked equally well for the closure of skin incisions and lacerations. A variety of smaller needles, designed for more specialized suturing, replaced the old and sizable finger-held needles that seemed more suitable for sewing a canvas sail than for the epidermis.

Efficient needle holders were distinguished by their short and powerful jaws with scored faces that could grip a needle securely. Generally a catch was necessary to keep the jaws clamped, and these ranged from earlier catch devices to none at all. Some of the more popular or interesting holders follow:

SLIDING HANDLE LOCK. c1880~1900

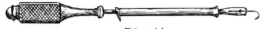

ROUX'S

AN ADAPTATION OF THE ANCIENT RING LOCK
(REYNDERS & CO. 1895)

RATCHET RELEASE CATCH.

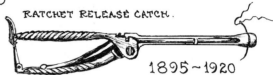

1895~1920

HAGEDORN'S
(REYNDERS 1915, KNY-SCHEERER 1915)

RATCHET RELEASE CATCH c 1895~1980's

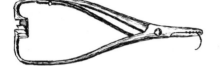

CROSBY-MATHIEU'S
(REYNDERS 1895~MILTEX 1973)

RATCHET RELEASE c.1915~1965

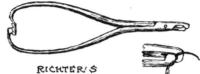

RICHTER'S
(REID 1915~WECK 1961)

RATCHET RELEASE c.1915~1950

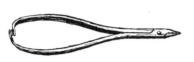

MURPHY'S
(REID 1915~ALOE 1947)

PIN + PINION CATCH c 1895~1920

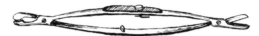

SKENE'S ~ DOUBLE-JAWED.
(REYNDERS 1895 ~ KNY-SCHEERER 1915)

NOTCHED HANDLE CATCHES ➤

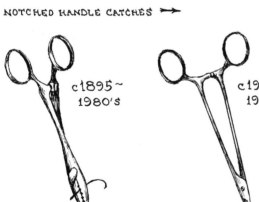

c1895~
1980's

ABBÉ'S
(REYNDERS 1895~MILTEX 1973)

c1910~
1980's

CRILE-MURRAY'S OR WOOD'S
(REID 1915 ~ MILTEX 1980's)

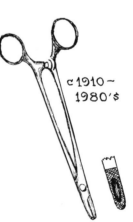

c1910~
1980's

MAYO-HEGAR'S
(REID 1915 ~ MILTEX 1980's)

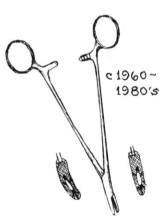

c1960~
1980's

METZENBAUM'S
(WECK 1961 ~ MILTEX 1980's)

NO CATCHES ➤

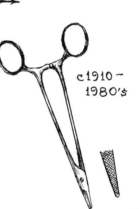

c1910~
1925

FOR INTESTINAL
SUTURING.

PRINTY'S
(REID 1915 ~ SHARP & SMITH 1925)

c1910~1975

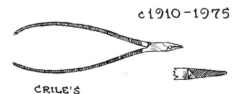

CRILE'S
(KNY-SCHEERER 1915~MILTEX 1973)

BULLET PROBES

The army surgeon had never seen the likes of bullet wounds before gunpowder was first used in the mid-thirteenth century. For the next three hundred years his treatment would rank high among the horrors of war. Since it was thought that the gunpowder itself was the irritant that caused wound inflammation, "neutralizers" were used as counterirritants. The unfortunate soldier was subjected to boiling hempseed oil or oil of violets being poured down the bullet's pathway. If hemorrhage complicated the wound, a red-hot cautery iron was plunged in to sear the ruptured artery. Any patient who survived such treatment received a bonus of a camphor or turpentine dressing.

There had to be a better way, and extracting the lead projectile became a priority in 1532 with the first screw retractor. Since hit-or-miss probing with the instrument only compounded bleeding and tissue damage, it became evident that first locating the bullet was a must.

In many cases, the surgeon's finger could locate the wayward sphere of lead. A female catheter or a metal rod could be put to service if the bullet had penetrated to greater depths. Most America texts up to the 1870's suggested such choices until the cause of wound contamination became known.

As for bullet probes, Scultetus made early mention of their use in his 1674 "Armamentarium." Contact with the bullet gave a feeling of roughness and resistance. A series of short jabs with the probe would yield a dull "thunk" and confirm the projectile's location.

By the Napoleonic Wars, the bullet probe was in general use. The ten to fifteen inch rods were often of silver, a more malleable metal that could be bent to pursue deflected musket balls. Each had a slightly bulbous end for surer contact and less tissue injury. Because the bullet forceps at the time were traumatic when opened, Savigny introduced a probe-forceps combination in the early nineteenth century. Hinged like midwifery forceps, the two parts could be separated, with one acting as a probe. When the bullet was located, the other blade was then inserted and the two locked together to secure the ball.

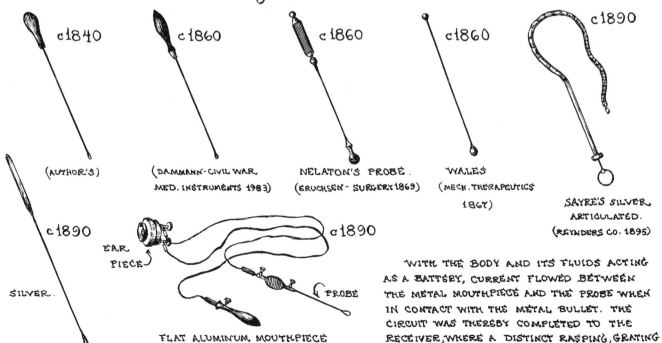

c1840 (AUTHOR'S)

c1860 (DAMMANN-CIVIL WAR MED. INSTRUMENTS 1983)

c1860 NELATON'S PROBE. (ERICHSEN - SURGERY 1869)

c1860 WALES (MECH. THERAPEUTICS 1867)

c1890 SAYRE'S SILVER ARTICULATED. (REYNDERS CO. 1895)

c1890 SILVER. BULLET PROBE (REYNDERS CO. 1895)

c1890 EAR PIECE PROBE FLAT ALUMINUM MOUTHPIECE DR. GIRDNER'S TELEPHONIC BULLET PROBE. (REYNDER'S CO. 1895)

WITH THE BODY AND ITS FLUIDS ACTING AS A BATTERY, CURRENT FLOWED BETWEEN THE METAL MOUTHPIECE AND THE PROBE WHEN IN CONTACT WITH THE METAL BULLET. THE CIRCUIT WAS THEREBY COMPLETED TO THE RECEIVER, WHERE A DISTINCT RASPING, GRATING OR CLICKING SOUND COULD BE HEARD.

BULLET EXTRACTORS

The screw extractor, the first instrument designed to remove bullets, first saw battlefield use in 1532. Its hollow, straight cylinder was pushed down the missile's path until the ball was contacted. An internal rod, tipped with a screw, was then rotated into the soft lead, secured for removal. This early extractor, admittedly along less ornate lines, was still in use before the First World War. However, it was rarely seen and used on this side of the Atlantic. Many of our nineteenth century writers called it worthless, perhaps because of the considerable tissue injury while attempting to impale a chunk of metal in the surrounding soft and yielding tissue.

c1535

(GERMANISCHES NATIONAL-MUSEUM, NUREMBERG)

Forceps were logical alternatives. Thompson, in his History of Surgical Instruments, mentions two such 1585 newcomers with blades serrated on the inside of the points for a better grip on the bullet. From the inventive mind of Ambroise Paré came both the Crane's Bill and Duck's Bill forceps. Probably both saw service in the Jamestown Colony before 1700.

1915

BAUDEN'S BULLET SCREW.

(KNY-SCHEERER CO. 1915)

c1585

PARÉ'S CRANE'S BILL FORCEPS,

FOR SMALL SHOT AND SPLINTERS OF ARMOR AND BONE IN DEEP WOUNDS.

PARÉ'S DUCK'S BILL FORCEPS FOR BULLETS IN DEEP FLESHY PARTS.

c1585

(THOMPSON-HISTORY OF SURGICAL INSTRUMENTS, 1941)

Alfonse Ferri of Naples perpetuated his name with the "Alfonsinum", a new application of the old ring lock. When the imbedded ball was contacted, the steel band was pulled back to its wooden handle to open the three steel prongs. A modest advancement of the instrument brought the teeth just beyond the target. The ring was then pushed down to close the teeth securely around the ball before extraction.

When the American Revolution erupted in 1775, any sort of medical and surgical supplies was almost non-existant. When Dr. Binney of the General Hospital was sent from the Army in New York to Philadelphia to purchase urgently needed instruments, he reported "...that there were no instruments to be purchased at any rate, and that the only workmen in the city that could make surgeons' instruments were engaged by Congress upon arms, and could not undertake any work for a long time to come." It seemed that there would be more musket balls flying than bullet forceps to retrieve them.

1590

EARLY 1600's

ALPHONSINE.
(THOMPSON - 1941)

MAGGIUS GOOSE-BILL
(SCULTETUS, 1674)

c1775

In 1776, it was recorded that the Regimental Surgeons of fifteen regiments surveyed had in their personal possession only four scalpels. In contrast to this incredible lack of the most basic of field instruments, there were "...three pair of forceps for extracting bullets." Certainly the removing of musket balls continued to be a high priority in the years ahead for the hard-pressed American physician.

Gunshot wounds on the battlefield often required amputation of a limb, especially if complicated by compound fractures of a limb or any joint penetration. English surgeon

AMERICAN BULLET FORCEPS.
(U.S. ARMY MEDICAL MUSEUM)

Richard Wiseman had championed this gradually accepted view back in the 1650's. To delay such surgery frequently meant overwhelming infection and death. (This was unfortunately so in the later Civil War period.)

Still, there was an increased emphasis on bathing, cleanliness of clothing and bedding, improved diet, and exercise in our Revolutionary war camps and hospitals. Dr. James Tilton, the sparkplug of these recommendations and healthful small fresh air hospital units, reported in 1778 "As to gunshot wounds, the only observation that occurs to me worth mentioning is, that the longer we continued in service, amputation and cutting became generally less fashionable. From obstinacy in the patients and other contingencies, we had frequent opportunities of observing that limbs might be saved which the best authorities directed to be cut off." Likely bacteria (although the germ infection theory was yet to be discovered) multiplied with less enthusiasm in a cleaner wound.

There were a number of different bullet extractors that followed the Revolutionary period.

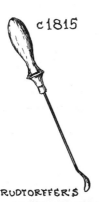

DR. JAMES TILTON
(1745~1822)

(WILBUR - REVOLUTIONARY MEDICINE 1700-1800, 1980)

MARKED "EVANS" OF LONDON, THESE FORCEPS WERE USED BY DR. CHRISTOPHER HEYDRICK.

(MUTTER MUSEUM, PHILADELPHIA)

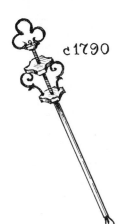

c1790

(DIDEROT'S ENCYCLOPEDIA, CHIRURGIE, PL. II 1790)

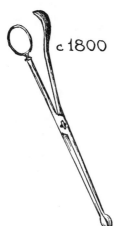

c1800

PERCY'S BULLET FORCEPS.
(SYNG, ELEMENTS SURGERY 1818)

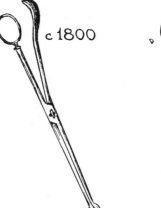

c1800

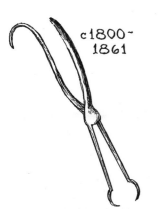

c1800~1861

OLD STYLE BULLET FORCEPS.
(GROSS-SYSTEM OF SURGERY 1862)

c1815

RUDTORFFER'S BULLET SCOOP (CONJECTURAL).
FIRST USED AS A PROBE, THEN BULLET SCOOPED OUT.
(THOMPSON - HIST. SURG. INST. 1941)

c1840~1870+

CONICAL, NOT ROUND BALLS MADE THE EUROPEAN VERSION PRACTICAL. AFTER THE SPOON TIP WAS PUSHED BEYOND THE BULLET, THE SCREW ROD WAS ADVANCED INTO THE BULLET.

KOLBE'S EXTRACTOR EXPANDED THE JAWS BY A SCREW IN THE HANDLE ONCE THE BULLET HAD BEEN CONTACTED.

c1850~1870±

EUROPEAN EXTRACTOR.
(ESP. BRITISH + FRENCH USAGE.
(GROSS - SYSTEM OF SURGERY VOL. I 1862)

KOLBE
AMERICAN

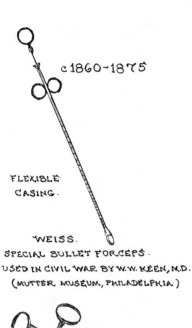

c 1860-1875

FLEXIBLE
CASING.

WEISS.
SPECIAL BULLET FORCEPS.
USED IN CIVIL WAR BY W.W. KEEN, M.D.
(MUTTER MUSEUM, PHILADELPHIA.)

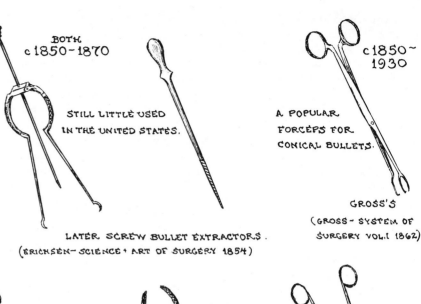

BOTH
c 1850-1870

STILL LITTLE USED
IN THE UNITED STATES.

LATER SCREW BULLET EXTRACTORS.
(ERICHSEN- SCIENCE + ART OF SURGERY 1854)

A POPULAR
FORCEPS FOR
CONICAL BULLETS.

GROSS'S
(GROSS- SYSTEM OF
SURGERY VOL.I 1862)

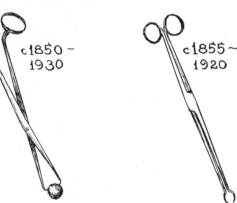

c 1850-
1930

TIEMANN'S FORCEPS.
(GROSS-SYSTEM OF SURGERY 1862)

c 1855-
1920

U.S. ARMY BULLET FORCEPS.
(MUTTER MUSEUM, PHILADELPHIA)

c 1855-
1920

U.S. ARMY BULLET FORCEPS
(DAMMANN- CIVIL WAR INST. 1983)

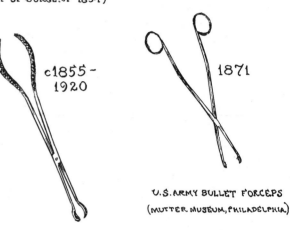

1871

U.S. ARMY BULLET FORCEPS
(MUTTER MUSEUM, PHILADELPHIA)

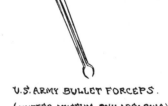

1876

BILL ARROWHEAD FORCEPS.
(THE MEDICAL RECORD 1876)

TIEMANN & CO.

There were several observations made by veteran surgeons concerning the extraction of musket balls. And foreign bodies driven down the bullet's path such as pieces of clothing, buttons and fragments of bone must be removed. Before searching for the ball, as Paré observed, that part of the body injured should be placed in the position when struck to better follow the path of the ball. (By the time of the Civil War, anesthetics were also useful by relaxing local muscle spasm) And good advice for those pre-sterilization surgeons-forget any search for the ball in the greater cavities of the body, for fatal internal injuries and increase infection risk must surely follow. Also, forget the screw bullet extractor- it's useless!

U.S. ARMY SURGEON T.H. BILL INVENTED THESE UNUSUAL FORCEPS FOR THE WESTERN INDIAN WARS. BILL SAID"...THAT FOR ARROWS NOT LODGED IN BONE THEY SHOULD BE INTRODUCED CLOSED, AND USED AS A SNARE BY WHICH THE IRON OR FLINT POINT OF THE ARROW MAY BE ENTANGLED. FOR AN ARROW LODGED, THEY ARE TO BE INTRODUCED CLOSED, CARRIED DOWN ALONG-SIDE THE FLAT SURFACE OF THE ARROW-HEAD, OPENED, AND THEN CLOSED ON THE FOREIGN BODY. "

INSTRUMENTS OF DESTRUCTION

Early on in America, the business of delivering babies was left to nature. The Reverend Johannes Megapolensis, Jr. made this clear in his 1644 <u>A Short Account of the Mohawk Indians</u>. "The women, when they have been delivered, go about immediately afterwards; and be it ever so cold, they wash themselves and the young child in the river or snow. They will not lie down (for they say that if they did they would soon die), but keep going about. They are obliged to cut wood, to travel three or four leagues with the child; in short, they walk, they stand, they work, as if they had not lain in, and we cannot see that they suffer any injury by it; and we sometimes try to purswade our wives to lie-in so, and that the way of lying-in in Holland is a mere fiddle-faddle!"

Although the average delivery could manage quite nicely without interference, there were exceptions. There might be an exhausted mother with inefficient contractions, a poorly positioned fetus such as in breech or transverse positions, maternal convulsions or hemorrhage, or a slightly constricted pelvis. It was then that forceps could improve an awkward presentation, and with gentle traction assure a happy "outcome."

Some pelvic contractures spelled disaster for the fetus ~ and frequently the mother. Dr. William Lusk, in his 1899 <u>The Science And Art Of Surgery</u> stated that "In our native American women abnormal pelves are rare" and that most country physicians had never encountered a case. It was not so in foreign countries, where German physicians, for example, found problem pelves in fourteen per cent of their deliveries. Rickets accounted for many such abnormalities. Before surgical sterility became the rule in the 1880's, Caesarian section was one of the most hazardous procedures. Fewer than half the mothers would survive their newly delivered infants."

WILBUR~NEW ENGLAND INDIANS, 1980.

PERFORATION ~ THE FIRST STEP OF THE CRANIOTOMY OPERATION. (LUSK~ SCIENCE AND ART OF SURGERY 1899)

There was an alternative, after considerable soul-searching. A hopelessly impacted fetus called for desperate measures if the mother's life were to be saved. The pre-Listerian answer was the craniotomy - the collapsing of the head to allow

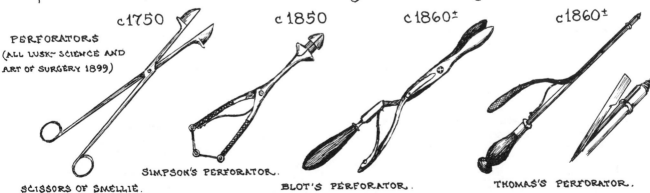

c1750   c1850   c1860±   c1860±

PERFORATORS (ALL LUSK~ SCIENCE AND ART OF SURGERY 1899)

SCISSORS OF SMELLIE.   SIMPSON'S PERFORATOR.   BLOT'S PERFORATOR.   THOMAS'S PERFORATOR.

TREPHINE PERFORATOR. ? DATE.
USED MOSTLY IN GERMANY, IT
REMOVED CIRCULAR SEGMENTS
OF SKULL TO LEAVE NO
SPLINTERS.
(LUSK~ SCIENCE AND
ART SURGERY 1899)

c1835
AMERICAN.

HODGE'S
CRANIOTOMY
SCISSORS ~ USED
AS A PERFORATOR
TO CUT AWAY PORTIONS
OF THE BONE.
(LUSK~ SURGERY 1899)

passage through the constricted pelvis. The perforator first bored an opening in the skull. The cranial bones were then separated by handle pressure and the brain tissue pulverized.

CROTCHET 1600's~1915.

The crotchet (French for small hook or crook) removed brain tissue and then used for traction after the head was perforated. Its sharp angled point could lacerate the pelvic passage and was little used after the coming of the cranio-clast (craniotomy forceps). Surprisingly, it and the other craniotomy instruments were still available in the Kny~Scheerer catalogue of 1915.

1600's ~ 1915
DR. TAYLOR'S RIGHT-
ANGLED BLUNT
HOOK.
(LUSK~1899)

The blunt hook, also from the seventeenth century, was chiefly used to apply traction to a part of the body of the fetus~particularly with a breech presentation.

FROM 1600's.

BOOM'S LEVER.
(RICCI~ GYN 1949)

TITSING'S LEVER.
(RICCI-DEVELOPMENT
GYN SURGERY AND
INSTRUMENTS 1942)

The seventeenth century lever was a strip of wood or metal with gently curved ends. It was used to pry the impacted head free from the pelvis, while no doubt causing considerable damage to the birth canal.

1740~1915

VECTIS
(KNY-SCHEERER
1915)

The vectis, invented in 1740, fortunately replaced the old lever. Basically half a forceps, it was likely a spin-off from Chapman's publication Obstetrics in 1733 when the mechanics of delivery forceps was first made public. The vectis could convert the impassable brow or shoulder positions to the normal vertex (top of the head) presentation.

The cephalotribe

The crotchet routinely followed the perforator until 1829. That year, before the prestigious Institut de France, Baudeloque underlined the dangers of using pointed and sharp-edged instruments in craniology and that half the mothers undergoing the procedure died. He then described his solution of the predicament; a two foot long cephalotribe that weighed over seven pounds and with two enormous blades that could crush the skull with a twist of the handle crank. Contrary to expectations, the perforator was still necessary to clear the brain tissue. The cephalotribe could then compress and apply traction to the head.

1829 ~ 1915

CEPHALOTRIBE OF
BLOT
(LUSK~ 1899)

c1870-15

SIMPSON'S
CRANIOCLAST.
(LUSK 1899)

The cranioclast, otherwise known as craniotomy forceps, was conceived by Sir J.Y Simpson to replace the cephalotribe. Basically a

powerful crusher and extractor, the larger fenestrated blade was positioned on the outer surface
of the head, while the smaller solid blade was
inserted into the previously perforated skull. The
crushed cranial vault was contained within the
scalp. Then traction could proceed with the
instrument.

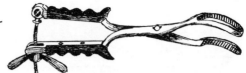

BRAUN'S CRANIOCLAST.
(LUSK-SCIENCE-ART SURGERY 1899)

Braun's modified cranioclast served as a tractor without crushing. The
head gradually molded to the pelvic axis with the help of the mother's contractions.
In this way, severe maternal lacerations and injuries were past history.
Fortunately, craniotomy soon thereafter also became history when aseptic
Caesarian sections safely changed the delivery route.

1554

OBSTETRICAL FORCEPS

Prior to the mid-eighteenth century, the lying-in chamber
was strictly a woman's domain. Poorly trained and with little more
than her experience to guide her, the midwife could manage the
uncomplicated delivery without much difficulty. The impacted
fetus was quite beyond her expertise, and if the mother were
to be saved, a surgeon would be called to perform the dreaded
craniotomy. Otherwise, the medical profession stood aloof from
the whole birth process, partly because of lack of knowledge,
and partly because the laying on of hands was felt beneath
his calling. There was the matter of female modesty as well.

RUEFF'S.
(MULDER/RICCI, 1949)

There were early efforts to assist the fetus in its travels through the
abnormal bony pelvic basin. Jacobus Rueff illustrated his 1554 treatise with
fixed pivot forceps. The concept worked better for splinters than babies. Because
both blades had to be introduced together, it was a near impossability to expand
them to enclose the head. Although their only use was for the extraction of
a dead fetus, it was a sorely needed beginning.

1720's ~ Dutch surgeon Jean Palfyn introduced a pair of spoon-shaped instruments without a
fixed pivot joint. Each could be passed separately
down the birth canal to enclose the fetal head.
But without any joint connection, the blades
lacked any pressure for traction.

1720's

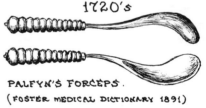

PALFYN'S FORCEPS.
(FOSTER MEDICAL DICTIONARY 1891)

c1730's

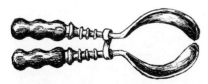

HEISTER TAPE ON PALFYN'S FORCEPS.
(RICCI-DEVELOPMENT OF GYN..., 1949)

HEISTER'S MOVABLE HOOK ON PALFYN'S.
(RICCI-DEVELOPMENT OF GYN..., 1949)

Professor Laurent Heister of Altdrof and Helmstadt
partially solved this problem once the spoons were
in place by joining the handles with a strap or
napkin. He later connected the spoons with a
mobile hook or ring collar that could slide up or
down the stems. In this way, the pressure on the
head could be adjusted.

As the search for more efficient obstetrical
forceps continued, it was rumored that a French
Huguenot family, transplanted to England, had discovered such an instrument. Indeed, Hugh Chamberlen
managed many difficult deliveries successfully, but
the method was a closely guarded secret. In 1688,
members of the Medico-Pharmaceutical College of
Amsterdam paid the Chamberlens a princely sum

for the device. They then ruled that no physician could practice midwifery without the secret instrument and a hefty financial consideration. The "secret" proved to be nothing more than a single bladed vectis. Canny son Hugh had sold but half of his father's invention!

Meanwhile the Chamberlens, with characteristic lack of altruism, passed the forceps from son to grandson. The family estate was sold in 1715, and just one hundred years later the lid was off the mystery~literally. A trap door was discovered in a closet floor, and underneath was a chest containing family momentos AND a number of those long~sought forceps. Rueff's earlier idea had been altered to fenestrated blades with a cephalic curve for a better hold on the fetal head. More important, the forceps could be separated and positioned before joining the blades at the pivot joint. The stems were then bound together with tape. The pivot lock was a vital part of this and all subsequent and successful forceps.

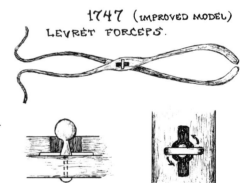

c 1660's

CEPHALIC CURVE

CHAMBERLEN'S FORCEPS ~ A SHORT INSTRUMENT WITH ONLY A CEPHALIC CURVE. (FOSTER MEDICAL DICTIONARY 1891)

The growing concern for better obstetrical treatment had not waited for the solution of the Chamberlen mystery. The Rueff and Palfyn contributions sparked renewed interest in the mechanisms of delivery. By the mid~eighteenth century, physicians had begun to replace the midwife. Thanks to the improved Palfyn, Levret and Smellie forceps, every mother~to~be could approach term with a far greater degree of confidence.

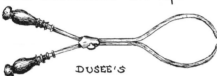

DUSEE'S IMPROVED PALFYN FORCEPS WITH SIMPLE SCREW LOCK. (RICCI ~ DEVELOPMENT OF GYN··· 1949)

1747~ Andre Levret of France gifted his forceps with several important improvements. The "French lock," refined by Dubois in 1791, was basically a revolving thumb lock that was inserted into a parallel slot, then turned to secure the blades into position. Levret also first added the pelvic curve to the earlier cephalic curve, assuring that not only the fetal head but also the perineum escaped injury.

1747 (IMPROVED MODEL) LEVRET FORCEPS.

PELVIC CURVE.

THE IMPROVED FRENCH LOCK. (LUSK ~ SCIENCE AND ART OF MIDWIFERY 1899)

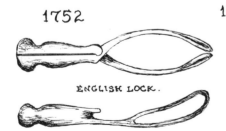

1752

ENGLISH LOCK.

SMELLIE'S FORCEPS. (RICCI ~ DEVELOPMENT GYN···, 1949)

1752~ English surgeon William Smellie's forceps contained the most advanced obstetrical pivot lock~ the "English lock." The notches in each stem fit together to lock the instrument~ convenient and efficient. Smellie, quite independent of Levret, also incorporated the pelvic curve into the blades. Of interest are the handle notches, a reminder of the early Palfyn handles that must be bound with tape to hold the blades together.

After well over two centuries, Smellie's forceps continue to be the most popular type in the British Empire.

1751~ John Burton's mechanical flop was described in his New System of Surgery. Burton had forgotten the importance of the pivot lock that allowed the blades to be introduced separately. Sir Alexander Simpson summed up this interesting also-ran as "…ingenious but very unserviceable, forceps working like a lobster's claw." The blades were unable to expand enough to enclose the head.

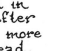

BUSCH'S FORCEPS.
(RICCI - DEVELOPMENT GYN…,1949)

1751

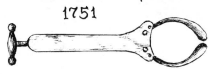

THE INTERNALS.

BURTON'S FORCEPS

(RICCI - DEVELOPMENT GYN…INST…,1949)

1793~ Obstetrical forceps are traction instruments. With this in mind, Johann Busch introduced finger rests for the first and second fingers. The Marlburg professor positioned these projections just below the pivot lock rather than the base of the handle to provide better axis traction. Busch also coated the blades with black rubber for better gripping.

1804 ~ E.C.J. von Siebold's completely new and efficient pivot lock captured the fancy of America's physicians. It was so well received that Dr. Hugh Hodge of Pennsylvania incorporated the lock in his 1833 model.

1812~ Robert P. James, a graduate of the University of Pennsylvania, deserves a place in history on several counts. When two veterans decided to use the Smellie's scissors and the crochet on a fetal head impaction, the attending women insisted on a consultation from Dr. James. Since he was but twenty years old, his elders ridiculed "the boy" being called in for an opinion. James not only disagreed~ he brought along forceps of his own design to prove his point. Shortly after, he delivered the child alive and kicking. As the word spread, forceps for impacted deliveries became more the rule rather than the exception.

1804

SCREW TO UNITE BLADES.   COUNTERSUNK FOR SCREW.
VON SIEBOLD'S FORCEPS.
(RICCI- DEVELOPMENT OF GYN SURGERY + INSTRUMENTS 1949)

The James forceps used the English lock. His narrow fenestrated blades were without beveling to better fit the fetal head for improved compression and traction.

1812

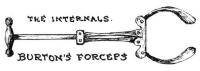

JAMES'S FORCEPS.
(RICCI- DEVELOPMENT GYN…,1949)

1825~ Using the English lock, David D. Davis, Professor of Midwifery at the University of London, introduced unequal blades for a poorly positioned head. The shorter blade was placed just behind the ear to act as a fulcrum.

1825

DAVIS'S ASYMMETRICAL.
(RICCI- DEVELOPMENT GYN…, 1949)

HODGE'S FORCEPS.
(LUSK-SCIENCE, ART OF MIDWIFERY 1899)

1833 ~ Pennsylvania's Hugh L. Hodge, in his Principles and Practice of Obstetrics described the French or Long forceps as those generally used in the United States. His own design, patterned after the French style, used Siebold's pivot lock. His more ovoid blades were less apt to slip from the head, and the parallel shanks with an increased pelvic curve prevented injury to the perineum.

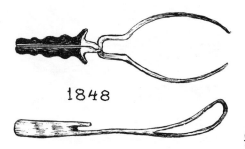

1848

SIMPSON'S FORCEPS.
(RICCI - DEVELOPMENT GYN··· 1949)

1848 ~ James Simpson, Professor of Obstetrics at Edinburgh, borrowed workable ideas from earlier instruments. Busch's finger rests were there, and he revived the deep finger depressions in the handle of Brunninghausen and Friess from the early nineteenth century. Incidentally, it was Simpson who first used ether in obstetrics January of 1847.

1853 ~ This was the German style lock, popular in that country but saw little service in the United States. The flattened head fit into a notch in the female stem for easy locking and separation.

1853

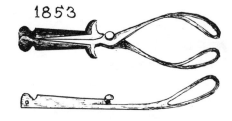

NAEGELE'S FORCEPS.
(LUSK-SCIENCE ART MIDWIFERY, 1899)

c 1865

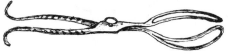

WALLACE'S FORCEPS.
(RICCI~DEVELOPMENT GYN··· INSTRUMENTS, 1949)

1865 ~ William Wallace, an English medical educator, moved to Brooklyn in 1864. His forceps with Davis blades and Hodges handles were light, easily joined and caused no injury to the mother or pressure marks on the child. Graduates of Jefferson Medical College were enthusiastic users of the forceps and were certainly popular elsewhere in the United States.

1858 ~ To prevent compression of the fetal head, Dr. George Elliot, Jr. of New York devised a sliding screw and pin on the inner surface of a handle. When joined, the pin kept the blades apart at the proper distance. This was a favorite in the New York area.

1858

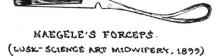

PIN →

ELLIOT'S FORCEPS.
(REYNDERS & CO. 1895)

1875

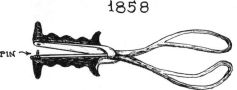

SMITH'S FORCEPS.
(RICCI-DEVELOPMENT GYN···, 1949)

1875 ~ Albert Holmes Smith, consulting obstetrician at the Philadelphia Hospital, modified the Davis forceps with a Siebold lock and both short and long separable handles. A pivot and ratchet made this interchange possible, depending on the degree compression necessary.

1877 ~ Two years earlier, Laroyenne had drilled holes in each blade where the center of the child's head would be held. Attached cords drew the head down the curved axis of the pelvis. Etienne Jarnier improved the concept with traction rods. While steady and easy traction was applied with the traction handle, the blades were free to turn in the axis of the pelvic cavity.

1877

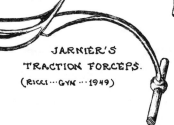

JARNIER'S TRACTION FORCEPS.
(RICCI···GYN···1949)

By the 1880's, obstetrical forceps were all metal for better sterilization. These later instruments borrowed the best from the past for a safer future.

SCISSORS

Generally, little notice is taken of the commonplace. Take scissors, for instance. There were few households in early America that could do without these instruments. Scissors were among the few medical necessities not urgently needed in the Revolutionary War. Few historical documents bothered to describe the obvious, but an idea of their changing designs may be gleaned from old title pages and surgical text drawings.

The Romans invented scissors by converting the tongs of the Egyptian type forceps into blades. Sheep shearers and grass clippers of recent memory testify to the usefulness of these spring blade closures. Tempered steel was produced by both the Greeks and Romans, although more intricate surgical instruments could be cast by combining copper and tin to make bronze. Probably both metals saw service in these early scissors.

The pivot-hinged blades in our modern scissors were certainly in use by the sixteenth century. Gross, in his 1862 <u>System of Surgery</u>, skims over the subject by saying "Scissors are nothing but two knives united by a screw, and furnished each with a ring-handle...." About this time Charrière, the famed Paris instrument maker, replaced the screw with a tenon pivot so that the blades could be separated for easier cleaning.

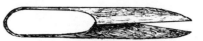

FIRST CENTURY B.C.
ROMAN SCISSORS.
(NATIONAL MUSEUM OF NAPLES)

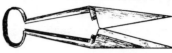

GREAT EASTERN SHEEP SHEARS.
(SEARS, ROEBUCK & CO., CHICAGO 1902)

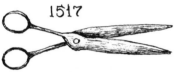

c1864
CHARRIÈRE'S TENON
PIVOT JOINT.

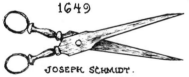

1517
(GERSDORFF 1517)

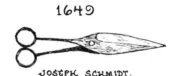

1500's
ARMY SURGEON'S SCISSORS.
(CIBA SYMPOSIA VOL I NO. 11 FEB. 1940)

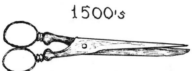

1634
AMBROSE PARÉ.
(GRAHAM- STORY OF SURGERY 1939)

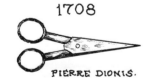

1649
JOSEPH SCHMIDT.
(INSTRUMENTA CHIRURGICA, AUGSBURG 1649)

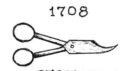

1649
JOSEPH SCHMIDT.
(INSTRUMENT CHIRURGICA, AUGSBURG 1649)

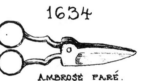

1708
PIERRE DIONIS.
(COURS D'OPÉRATIONS DE CHIRURGIE, PARIS, 1708)
POSSIBLY EARLY BANDAGE SCISSORS.

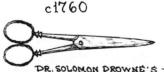

1708
PIERRE DIONIS.
(COURS D'OPÉRATIONS DE CHIRURGIE 1708)

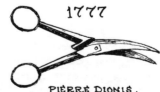

1708
PIERRE DIONIS.
(COURS D'OPÉRATIONS DE CHIRURGIE, PARIS 1708)

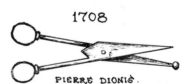

c 1765~1781
DICTIONNAIRE DES SCIENCES.
(PLANCHES TOME II, 1781)

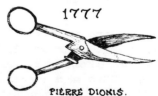

c1760
DR. SOLOMON DROWNE'S -
CONTINENTAL ARMY SURGEON.
(ARMED FORCES INST. OF PATHOLOGY)

1777
PIERRE DIONIS.
(COURS D'OPÉRATIONS DE CHIRURGIE, PARIS, 1777)

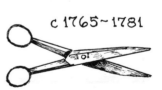

1777
PIERRE DIONIS.
(COURS D'OPÉRATIONS DE CHIRURGIE, 1777)

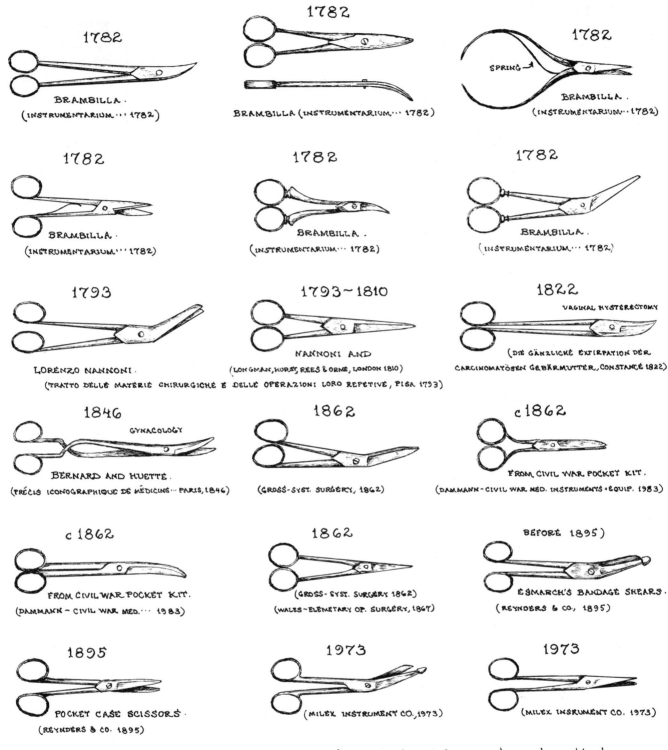

1782 BRAMBILLA. (INSTRUMENTARIUM ··· 1782)

1782 BRAMBILLA (INSTRUMENTARIUM ··· 1782)

1782 SPRING BRAMBILLA. (INSTRUMENTARIUM ··· 1782)

1782 BRAMBILLA. (INSTRUMENTARIUM ··· 1782)

1782 BRAMBILLA. (INSTRUMENTARIUM ··· 1782)

1782 BRAMBILLA. (INSTRUMENTARIUM ··· 1782)

1793 LORENZO NANNONI. (TRATTO DELLE MATERIE CHIRURGICHE E DELLE OPERAZIONI LORO REPETIVE, PISA 1793)

1793~1810 NANNONI AND (LONGMAN, HURST, REES & ORME, LONDON 1810)

1822 VAGINAL HYSTERECTOMY (DIE GÄNZLICHE EXTIRPATION DER CARCINOMATÖSEN GEBÄRMUTTER, CONSTANCE 1822)

1846 GYNACOLOGY BERNARD AND HUETTE. (PRÉCIS ICONOGRAPHIQUE DE MÉDICINE ··· PARIS, 1846)

1862 (GROSS-SYST. SURGERY, 1862)

c 1862 FROM CIVIL WAR POCKET KIT. (DAMMANN ~ CIVIL WAR MED. INSTRUMENTS + EQUIP. 1983)

c 1862 FROM CIVIL WAR POCKET KIT. (DAMMANN ~ CIVIL WAR MED. ··· 1983)

1862 (GROSS- SYST. SURGERY 1862) (WALES~ELEMETARY OP. SURGERY, 1867)

BEFORE 1895) ESMARCH'S BANDAGE SHEARS. (REYNDERS & CO., 1895)

1895 POCKET CASE SCISSORS. (REYNDERS & CO. 1895)

1973 (MILEX INSTRUMENT CO., 1973)

1973 (MILEX INSTRUMENT CO. 1973)

Although there was a trend toward simplicity of design, it is clear that scissors changed little through the centuries. As for function, straight scissors were used for dissecting, dressings and bandages. Those curved on the flat conveniently removed skin growths and were helpful in cavities where straight blades would injure the tissues. Angular scissors ~ those curved on their edges ~ divided tissues raised on a director or opening fistulas. Their angularity kept the blades parallel to the skin. Those with a knob at the end of one blade could remove bandages without the skin getting nicked.

DIRECTOR.

SCALPELS ~ (Latin scalpellus - a small, light surgical knife)

Several thousand years have passed since the Hindus forged the first known scalpels for incising, extracting foreign bodies, scarifying and drawing of bodily fluids. It's likely that the Greek surgeons continued these practices with like instruments, but any evidence of their steel specimens have long since rusted into nothingness. Our first inkling of their design comes from a time-resistant stone tablet found at the Athens Acropolis.

Each double-ended specimen had both blade and spatula (cased in alternating positions). The "bellied" blades, Greek meaning "like a breast of a woman," were apparently used to incise the skin between the ribs. All blades were crafted of tempered steel, as were the spatulas at the opposite end that were used for blunt tissue dissection. This double-ended arrangement, with modifications, was valued up to our twentieth century.

BAS-RELIEF OF SURGICAL CASE FROM THE ASCLEPIAION OF ATHENS. (MUSEUM OF ATHENS, GREECE)

The Romans continued the steel double-ended tradition to some degree, but fortunately for our study, bronze was the preferred metal. Here was an admirable alloy that could be cast into intricate shapes, took a fine polish AND never disappeared into a powder of ferric oxide.

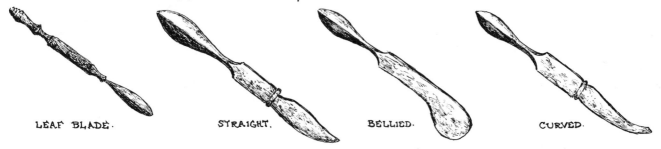

LEAF BLADE.   STRAIGHT.   BELLIED.   CURVED.

FIRST CENTURY B.C. BRONZE SCALPELS FOUND AT POMPEII. (NATIONAL MUSEUM OF NAPLES)

Our modern scalpels had their beginnings with the Roman single-ended instrument. The blade was attached to the handle with a thread or wire and could be removed for cleaning. As for the handles, they were generally round, square or hexagonal in cross-section.

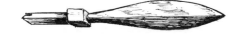

DETACHABLE BRONZE LEAF BLADE.
FIRST CENTURY B.C. BRONZE   STRAIGHT BLADE.
(VÉDRÈNES~TRAITÉ DE MEDICINE ···, PARIS, 1876 ~ RICCI)

The bleak middle ages, sandwiched between Antiquity and the Renaissance (A.D. 476 ~ A.D. 1453) offered nothing to the advancement of medicine, or anything else for that matter. Thereafter, the pocket scalpel began its long career that lasted into our present century. Because the blade folded into the handle, they could be carried protected and sharp ~ and one's pocket remained intact. France's famed surgeon

1497

FOLDING SCALPEL.
(BRUMSCHWIG~CHIRURGIA, 1497)

Ambroise Paré carried a pocket scalpel with a handle embellished with a winged figure of a woman, something of a work of art. Even advanced antique instrument collectors have overlooked what appeared to be an early jack knife.

1500s. The blades were usually leaf-shaped with double cutting edges and were riveted to a handle of wood or bone.

1598   1598

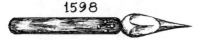

LEAF BLADE SCALPEL.   DOUBLE-ENDED BELLIED.   IT TOOK A VERY CAREFUL

(GUILLEMEAU, 1598 ~ FROM THOMPSON)   (DELLA CROCE, 1597 ~ FROM THOMPSON)   SURGEON TO MANAGE THIS ONE!

1600s. Here was a return to all-metal scalpels with an emphasis on curved blades.

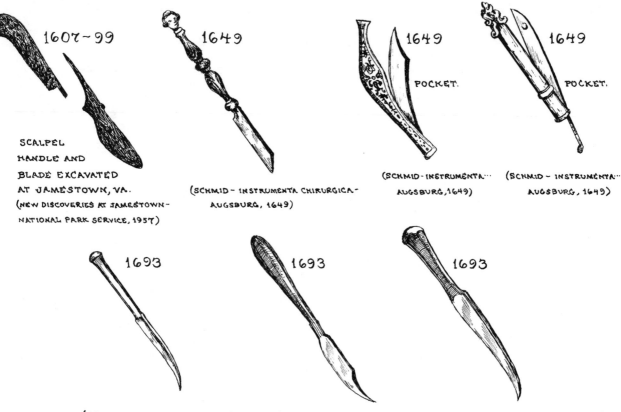

1607~99

SCALPEL HANDLE AND BLADE EXCAVATED AT JAMESTOWN, VA.
(NEW DISCOVERIES AT JAMESTOWN ~ NATIONAL PARK SERVICE, 1957)

1649
(SCHMID ~ INSTRUMENTA CHIRURGICA ~ AUGSBURG, 1649)

1649   POCKET.
(SCHMID ~ INSTRUMENTA ~ AUGSBURG, 1649)

1649   POCKET.
(SCHMID ~ INSTRUMENTA ~ AUGSBURG, 1649)

1693   1693   1693

(SCALPELS ILLUSTRATED BY SCULTETUS ~ ARMAMENTARIUM CHIRURGICUM, LEYDEN, 1693)

1700s. Pocket scalpels became increasingly popular from the beginning of the century with a preference for curved blades that folded into tortoise shell handles.

Leaf-shaped fixed blades of the period had single cutting edges. Blades were riveted to wood, bone or ivory handles.

1708   POCKET.   1708   POCKET.   1708   POCKET.

(DIONIS ~ COURS D'OPÉRATIONS DE CHIRURGIE, PARIS, 1708)

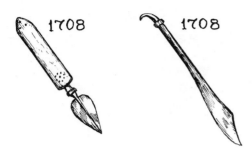

1708   1708

By the last quarter of the century, the leaf-shaped blades once again had double cutting edges. All blades were secured to the handles with a metal collar.

    Handles showed the greatest change. Of ivory, bone or checkered wood, they ended in a fan-shaped spatula. As a modified double-ended scalpel, the handle itself was used for blunt dissection.

(DIONIS - COURS D'OPÉRATIONS DE CHIRURGIE, PARIS, 1708)

LATE 1700s.

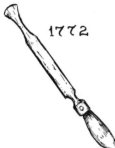

1772

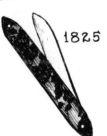

c1776

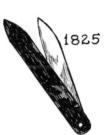

1777

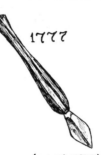

1782

(PERRET - 1772)   (WILBUR - REV. MEDICINE 1980)   (DIONIS - COURS··· 1777)

BRAMBILLA - INSTRU · CHIRURG · MILITARE ··· VIENNA, 1782)

1800s. Early on, the scalpel had become simplified into a handsome and efficient cutting instrument. The tortoise shell pocket scalpels, relatively unchanged throughout the eighteenth century, became less curved, carried a less pronounced curl to the tail, and lost the fancy rosette rivets in favor of simple rod rivets. By the 1820's the handle ends resembled a flat torpedo, then became rounded prior to the Civil War. The 1850's introduced the double-bladed pocket scalpel—a boon for reducing the bulk carried in the pocket case.

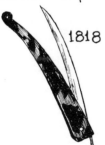

1818

1825   1825

COCKING PIN.

c 1850+

(DORSEY-ELEMENTS SURGERY, 1818)   (HISTORICAL MUSEUM MEDICINE + DENTISTRY, HARTFORD)   (WALES – ELEMENTARY OPERATIONS IN SURGERY, 1867)

    Fixed scalpel blades became shorter and straight or slightly curved. Their tangs were riveted to thin and flat ivory handles. The fan-shaped spatula end gradually became less pronounced. Hardwood handles such as ebony were popular by the Civil War and were often scored or checkered for a better grasp. By this period the handles had become more bulbous while the spatula and was little more than vestigial. The modern all-metal scalpel came into its own by the 1880's, free of bacteria and artistic appeal.

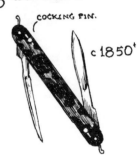

c 1800+

IVORY HANDLE.

SIR WILLIAM FERGUSSON'S

(THOMPSON - HIST + EVOL. SURG. INST. 1941)

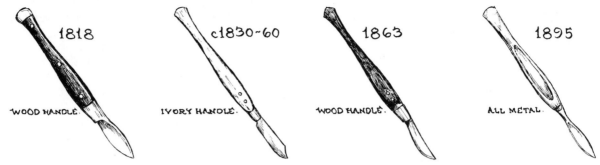

1818 — WOOD HANDLE.

c1830~60 — IVORY HANDLE.

1863 — WOOD HANDLE.

1895 — ALL METAL.

(DORSEY-ELEMENTS OF SURGERY, 1818)   (CAMMANK - CIVIL WAR INST··· 1983)   (SMITH - P.+R SURGERY 1863)   (REYNDERS & CO. 1895)

1900s. The basic scalpel design really hasn't changed since the all metal version of the late 1800's. But the age of throw-aways was upon us by 1925. Sharp and Smith broke the renewable B-R-X news with this 1925 flyer. That same year Frank S. Betz Company offered the Bard Parker. The 1927 Sharp and Smith catalogue no longer carried the B-R-X, but opted for the Bard Parker ~ very much in use to this day.   1925

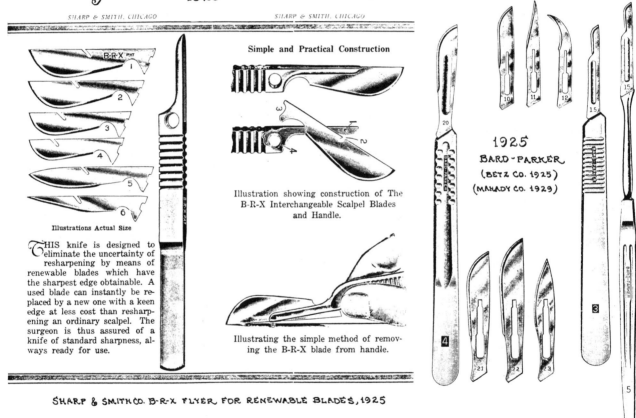

SHARP & SMITH, CHICAGO   SHARP & SMITH, CHICAGO

B-R-X PAT
1 2 3 4 5 6

Illustrations Actual Size

THIS knife is designed to eliminate the uncertainty of resharpening by means of renewable blades which have the sharpest edge obtainable. A used blade can instantly be replaced by a new one with a keen edge at less cost than resharpening an ordinary scalpel. The surgeon is thus assured of a knife of standard sharpness, always ready for use.

Simple and Practical Construction

Illustration showing construction of The B-R-X Interchangeable Scalpel Blades and Handle.

Illustrating the simple method of removing the B-R-X blade from handle.

1925
BARD - PARKER
(BETZ CO. 1925)
(MAHADY CO. 1929)

SHARP & SMITH CO. B-R-X FLYER FOR RENEWABLE BLADES, 1925

HOLDING THE SCALPEL ~ If the surgeon held his pen correctly when writing prescriptions, were skillful at the dining table with his steak knife, and could play the violin reasonably well, he was prepared for the basic scalpel incisions. There were four positions:

1. The pen-holding position for quick, delicate and precise cutting, here was a favorite. It was used for many operations such as lithotomy, excision of tumors, herniotomy and the extraction of cataracts.

(GROSS ~ SYSTEM OF SURGERY, 1862)

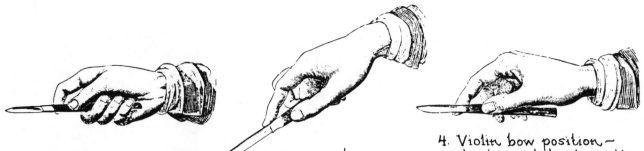

2. Common carving knife position.

3. A second carving knife position.

4. Violin bow position — used where delicate cutting is necessary.

2. and 3. used when force and firmness needed.

BISTOURIES — (probably named for the town of Pistori where a great plenty of these instruments were made.) They differed from the ordinary scalpel by being longer and more slender. There were many varieties: straight or curved blades, blunt or sharp points, and fixed handles or folding blades.

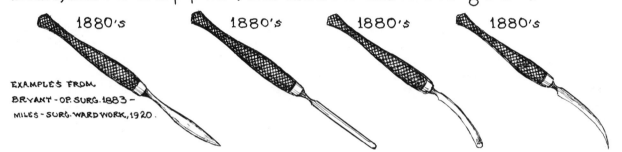

1880's   1880's   1880's   1880's

EXAMPLES FROM BRYANT - OP. SURG. 1883 - MILES - SURG. WARD WORK, 1920.

STRAIGHT SHARP-POINTED BISTOURY.   STRAIGHT PROBE-POINTED.   CURVED PROBE-POINTED.   CURVED SHARP-POINTED.

Among the bistouries' many uses were incisions through the abdominal wall where the thickness of tissue is considerable, in laying open sinuses, and in small amputations such as of fingers or toes.

For irriducible or strangulated hernias, a special curved blunt-pointed bistoury was introduced in the early 1800's. A short cutting edge in the blade's curve permitted division of the stricture without injuring the surrounding tissues.

c1810

CUTTING EDGE

ASTLY COOPER'S HERNIA BISTOURY.
(DORSEY - ELEMENTS OF SURGERY, 1818)

When handling these early instruments, there are moments when one ponders the successes and failures of the former owner. And speaking of strangulated hernias, it's hard to forget a turn-of-the century adventure of a fellow Vermont College of Medicine physician. It's worth repeating.

In his Memoirs Of A Small Town Surgeon, Dr. John Wheeler tells of a hurried train ride to North Ferrisburg. From there it was a two hour sleigh ride through two feet of snow to reach the patient. The strangulated hernia was ripe and the only operating table was a double bed that crowded out all but a two-foot space beside it. Wheeler's light was a kerosene lamp — to be held by a volunteer standing in the one-foot space at the foot of the bed.

"There was a little hesitation at first, but soon a hero stepped forward, remarking that he never see nobody bootchered and he'd kinder like to see haow they done it. He took his position at the foot of the bed, holding the lamp, and I began operating.

Hernia operations are not very bloody ones, but of course there is some bleeding, and as soon as the sponges began to look a little gory, the torch-bearer suddenly said 'Gosh! I got ter hev some air !' He thrust the lamp into the hands of a fellow who was looking in the door and rushed out of the house. No. Two stood to his guns pretty well, but when No. One returned and pluckily demanded the lamp, No. Two handed it back to him without any manifestations of reluctance. But in a few minutes No. One wilted again and beat another hasty retreat. Back he came, with renewed courage (and real courage it was), and took the lamp once more. This time he didn't wilt, but misfortune still attended him. I had just introduced the knife into the opening whose edges were compressing and strangulating the hernia, and according to the technique of the period I was very cautiously beginning to cut through the constriction—when things happened. No. One in his anxiety to give me as much light as possible, leaned forward over the bed and held the lamp out as near to me as he could. The etherizer became so interested in the operation that he failed to keep his patient completely unconcious. Consequently, at the most critical moment of the whole operation, the patient gave a kick. His knees struck the hand that was holding the lamp. Fortunately, the lamp was not knocked out of the hand, but the the chimney was knocked off the lamp, the lamp went out, and I was in total darkness, holding a knife whose point was in the abdominal cavity of a squirming half-concious patient. I made a somewhat peremptory demand for another lamp and a woman hurried in with the only other lamp in the house. By the light, the holder of the extinguished lamp saw his chimney lying on the bed and grabbed it. As it was almost hot enough to scorch the bed clothes, he dropped it with a yell and again rushed out of the house. I could hear him under the window, trying to cool off in the snow and inquiring for Helen Blazes. As the lady gave no evidence of hearing him, it seems probable that she was not within half a mile of the house.

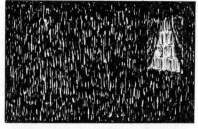

VIEW OF DR. WHEELER'S SURGERY.

The rest of the operation was uneventful."

OTHER SPECIALIZED SCALPELS ~

As one might suspect, the short-bladed scalpel had many such specialized offshoots. Some will be considered in later pages with their special operations. Others include the gum"lancet" with its curved cutting blade aslant from its narrow stem. Its use is obvious.

Probably the curved sharp-pointed multi-use scalpel was the forerunner of the sturdy abscess "lancet".

1867

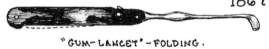

"GUM-LANCET"~FOLDING.
(WALES-ELEMENTARY OPERATIONS IN SURGERY, 1867)

1867

SYME'S "ABSCESS LANCET
(WALES- ELEMENTARY OP. SURGERY, 1867)

Although known as lancets, by definition they were not.

Tenotomes were small-bladed scapula that were used in tonectomy. To correct a deformity that resulted from muscular contraction, the blade was inserted on the flat and close to the tendon. The edge of the blade was then turned and the tendon severed with a sawing motion. The procedure gradually fell from favor as antiseptic surgery became popular. Open division was much to be preferred instead of blind cutting.

1902

(BRYANT ~ OPERATIVE
SURGERY, 1902)

VARIOUS
TENOTOME BLADES.

BLOODLETTING INSTRUMENTS

The practice of phlebotomy (Greek phlebos = vein and temnein = to cut) seemed logical enough when the foundation of treatment was based on the bodily humors; blood, phlegm, yellow bile and black bile. Excessive humors were believed to cause such symptoms as fever and inflammation. (By the mid-eighteenth century, excessive nerve stimulation was considered the exciting cause of disease. Purging, starving, vomiting or bloodletting would rid the patient of this over-abundance and health should be just a lancet-puncture away.

The art of phlebotomy was flourishing well before Hippocrates' fifth century B.C. By the middle ages, both surgeons and barbers were specializing in this bloody bonanza. Through the centuries the latter advertized with a red (for the blood let) and a white (for the tourniquet and the bandage that stemmed the bleeding) stripe pole (representing the stick held by the patient to dilate the veins).

Bloodletting came to America on the Mayflower. Samuel Fuller, a passenger without benefit of a medical certificate, wrote to Governor Bradford on June 28, 1630 that "I have been to Matapan [Dorchester] and let some twenty of those people blood. What disease prevailed among those people that required the loss of blood in the warm season of June, we are unable to determine."

1628

WILLIAM HARVEY'S "FOREARM VEINS.
(EXERCITATIO ANATOMICA DU MOTU CORTIS ET SANGUINIS ... FRANKFORT 1628)

Further south, the secretary and recorder of Jamestown Colony, William Strachey wrote "... there being at first but few physique helps, or skillfull surgeons who knew how to apply the right medicine in a new country, or to search the quality and constitucion of the patient, and his distemper, or that knew how to councell, when to lett blood, or not, or in necessity to use a launce in that office at all."

The practice reached unbelievable heights in the eighteenth and early nineteenth centuries. Dr. Benjamin Rush didn't hesitate to remove a quart of blood every forty-eight hours, and George Washington passed on to his reward with a throat infection, and without the nine pints of blood that was let in twenty-four hours!

By the War of 1812, surgeon James Mann was recording the up-to-date view that "... the more blood expended the better in wounds of the viscera, provided life is not exhausted, when haemorrhage is stopped." He went on to say that "it is good practice to bleed in all cases of wounds by musket balls, or bayonet, where there is but little loss of blood from the wound."

G. WASHINGTON in his last Illngs attended by Doc.rs Craik and Brown

ETCHING, PEMBER & LUZARDER, PHILADELPHIA, 1800.
(NEW YORK HISTORICAL SOCIETY, NEW YORK.)

Thereafter, phlebotomy gradually lost favor. Only apoplexy, pneumonia, poly-cythemia, pulmonary edema and congestive cardiac failure were considered treatable in this way. By the last quarter of the nineteenth century, Oliver Wendell Holmes summed up the all but obsolete treatment when he remarked that "The lancet was the magician's wand of the dark ages of medicine."

Before it became an embarrassment to the medical community, blood excesses were removed by two methods:

1. GENERAL PHLEBOTOMY required a lancet for the greatest venous (and arterial) yield
2. LOCAL BLOODLETTING drained swollen surface capillaries of their inflammation by scarification, cupping and leeching.

LANCETS ~ A surgical knife with a short, wide, pointed double-edged blade. Preferred general phlebotomy sites were the back of the hand, arm, ankle, jugular and frontal veins, as well as those under the tongue. Obviously, there were many alternatives, all of which the various bloodletting charts left no doubt.

After a promising puncture site was selected, a tape tourniquet was tied above and toward the heart while the operator's thumb temporarily compressed the vessel just below. With the engorged vein an easy target, the lancet blade made an incision of about a fifth of an inch, slightly oblique to the axis of the vein. An assistant caught the stream of blood in a shallow flat-bottomed bowl.

When the proper amount of blood was let, pressure over the incision usually controlled further bleeding.

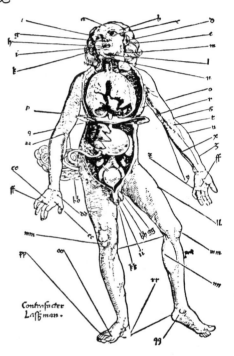

BLOODLETTING CHART (JOHANNES WECHTLIN)

A FEW PORRINGERS WERE MARKED WITH INNER RINGS FOR MEASURING THE YIELD. IN AMERICA, PROBABLY ANY HANDY HOUSEHOLD BOWL WAS PRESSED INTO SERVICE. THERE IS NO EVIDENCE THAT BARBER BOWLS WITH A SEMICIRCLE CUT OUT OF ITS WIDE RIM FOR THE NECK, WERE EVER USED IN BLOODLETTING.

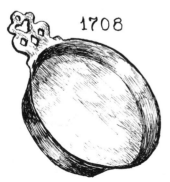

1607~1699

CERAMIC BLEEDING BOWL EXCAVATED AT JAMESTOWN, VA.
(HUDSON - NEW DISCOVERIES AT JAMESTOWN, NATIONAL PARK SERVICE, 1957)

1708

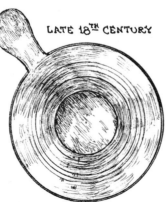

LATE 18TH CENTURY

BLOOD BASIN.
(DIONIS-COURS D'OPERATIONS DE CHIRURGIE, 1708)

PEWTER BLEEDING BOWL.
(SMITHSONIAN)

c.1750

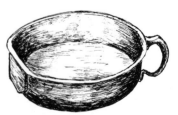

PEWTER BLEEDING BOWL.
(HUGH MERCER'S APOTHECARY, FREDERICKSBURG, VIRGINIA)

Four types of lancets served the phlebotomist through the centuries, all with the sharp-pointed, double-edged and straight blades necessary for a controlled vein puncture. They were the scalpel lancet, fleam, thumb and spring lancet.

SCALPEL LANCET

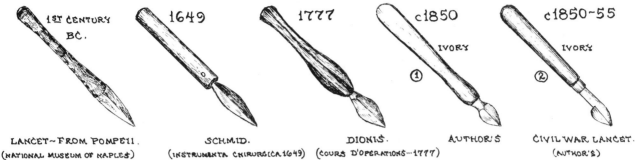

1st CENTURY BC.
LANCET~FROM POMPEII.
(NATIONAL MUSEUM OF NAPLES)

1649
SCHMID.
(INSTRUMENTA CHIRURGICA-1649)

1777
DIONIS.
(COURS D'OPERATIONS...1777)

c1850 IVORY ①
AUTHOR'S

c1850~55 IVORY ②
CIVIL WAR LANCET.
(AUTHOR'S)

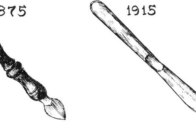

c1865 EBONY ③
AUTHOR'S.

c1875 ④
VICTORIAN LANCET.
(SMITHSONIAN ~ DAVIS)

1915
"THUMB LANCET" ALL METAL
(KNY SCHEERER CO. 1915)

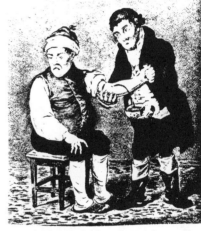

"BREATHING A VEIN."
(GILLRAY CARTOON ~ LITHOGRAPH, LONDON 1804)

A MINOR MYSTERY~ Many an antiques dealer (and Sears, Roebuck Catalogue of 1906!) will tell you that ① through ④ are "Steel Ink Erasers and Envelope Opener." It is difficult to understand why one would scuff up a mistake on paper in 1906 or try to open an envelope with such a short, curved double-edged blade. Perhaps, as Lister's surgical sterilization revolution gained momentum in the 1880's, horn, ivory and wooden-handled lancets became obsolete surplus on the retailers' shelves. And after some head-scratching, less surgical uses were invented. At any rate, these specimens would seem to fit the lancet definition.

FLEAM ~ A wide double-edged blade at right angles to the handle.

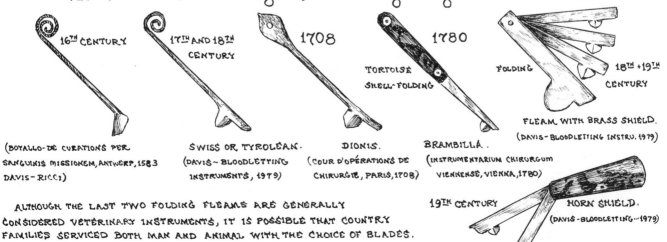

16TH CENTURY
(BOYALLO-DE CURATIONS PER SANGUINIS MISSIONEM, ANTWERP, 1583 DAVIS-RICCI)

17TH AND 18TH CENTURY
SWISS OR TYROLEAN.
(DAVIS ~ BLOODLETTING INSTRUMENTS, 1979)

1708
DIONIS.
(COUR D'OPÉRATIONS DE CHIRURGIE, PARIS, 1708)

1780
TORTOISE SHELL-FOLDING
BRAMBILLA.
(INSTRUMENTARIUM CHIRURGUM VIENNENSE, VIENNA, 1780)

FOLDING **18TH + 19TH CENTURY**
FLEAM WITH BRASS SHIELD.
(DAVIS-BLOODLETTING INSTRU. 1979)

19TH CENTURY
HORN SHIELD.
(DAVIS ~ BLOODLETTING...1979)

ALTHOUGH THE LAST TWO FOLDING FLEAMS ARE GENERALLY CONSIDERED VETERINARY INSTRUMENTS, IT IS POSSIBLE THAT COUNTRY FAMILIES SERVICED BOTH MAN AND ANIMAL WITH THE CHOICE OF BLADES.

THUMB LANCET ~ Introduced about the fifteenth century, the double-edged blade could be pivoted between the horn or tortoise shell handles. With thumb pressure, the blade could be positioned at any angle for the thrust.

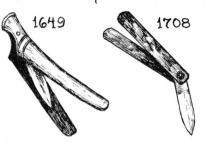

1649

1708

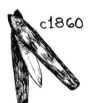

1793

(NANNONI - TRATTATO DEL MATERIE
CHIRURGICHE ··· PISA, 1793)

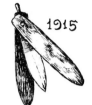

c1860

1915

(DAVIS- BLOODLETTING
INSTRUMENTS, 1979)

(KNY-SCHEERER CO., N.Y., 1915)

(SCHMID-INSTRUMENTA
CHIRURGICA, AUGSBURG, 1649)

(DIONIS-COURS DE OPÉRATIONS
DE CHIRURGIE, PARIS, 1708)

~THUMB LANCETS CHANGED LITTLE THROUGH THE CENTURIES~

SPRING LANCET ~ The idea came from Germany and was first described by Heister in 1719. Basically, it was a fleam that was snapped into the vein with a spring. It was a tiny instrument. The case was about $1\frac{5}{8} \times \frac{5}{8}$ inches (4 x 1.5 cm) and made of copper, brass, silver or an alloy. It was a favorite bloodletter in Germany, Holland and America, while the French and British continued with the older thumb lancet. Although the spring lancet required considerably less skill, it was a difficult instrument to clean and was a self-contained home for assorted bacteria.

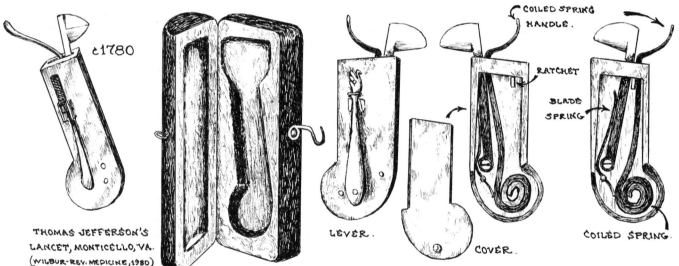

c1780

COILED SPRING
HANDLE.

RATCHET

BLADE
SPRING

THOMAS JEFFERSON'S
LANCET, MONTICELLO, VA.
(WILBUR-REV. MEDICINE, 1980)

LEVER.

COVER.

COILED SPRING.

LEATHER-COVERED AND LINED WOODEN CASE WITH BRASS FLEAM AND STEEL WORKINGS.

ARMING THE SPRING LANCET ~ PROJECTING FROM THE UNDERSIDE OF THE SHORT ARM OF THE LEVER WAS THE LANCET. THIS FLATTENED AS THE HANDLE OF THE COILED SPRING WAS PULLED BACK, THEN RETURNED TO POSITION TO CATCH THE COCKED SPRING. THE BLADE SHAFT WAS ALSO FORCED BACKWARD BY ITS LIGHTER SPRING. WHEN THE LONG ARM OF THE LEVER WAS PRESSED, THE SHORT ARM AND ITS RATCHET WERE RAISED TO RELEASE THE COILED SPRING. THE BLADE WAS SENT PLUNGING INTO THE VEIN.

The letting of blood was usually enthusiastic~ sixteen to thirty ounces were the average for anyone in "bad humor." As a rule of thumb, bleeding was continued to the point of faintness. The patient's flushed skin had become pallid, the hard and bounding pulse of ninety to one hundred and twenty beats per minute was now feeble, the fever had cooled, and the restlessness was replaced with a shock-like state. In theory it all seemed beneficial, and all it took was ten percent or more blood loss to be rid of the "excesses" causing illness. But with just six quarts of blood in the average patient's possession before lancing, the victim must face his illness with his bodily defenses lost to the bleeding bowl.

LOCAL BLOOD DEPLETION ~ CUPPING

Cupping was an adjunct to general phlebotomy - a way to bring an excessive concentration of blood to the skin from deeper problem sites. A heated cup of flint glass, or perhaps one of tin or horn, drew up the congestion by creating a vacuum on the skin as the hot air cooled. The skin became reddened and swollen inside the cup. With this evidence that the bad blood had surfaced, the vacuum was relieved by tilting the cup and gently pressing the skin away from the thick rim. Likely cupping had its origins in the practice of sucking up blood from poisoned wounds. Indeed, some cupping devices did use mouth suction rather than heat to evacuate the inner air. Like general phlebotomy, cupping was an ancient practice that enjoyed a surge of popularity in the seventeenth, eighteenth and nineteenth centuries.

The Greeks and Romans favored metal cups as did later military surgeons for their sturdiness in the field. Brass and pewter were common in the seventeeth and on through the nineteenth century. Slightly domed pressed horn cups, light to carry and often nested in sets of three, saw service in the first half of the nineteenth century ~ perhaps before.

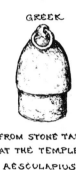

GREEK

FROM STONE TABLET
AT THE TEMPLE OF
AESCULAPIUS.

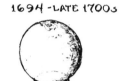

1694 -LATE 1700s

BLOWN GLASS
(DEKKERS~
EXERCITATIONES
PRACTICAE ··· 1694)

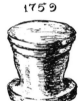

1759

? BRASS
(HEISTER~
GENERAL SYSTEM
OF SURGERY. 1759)

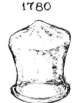

1700s ~1800s

PEWTER
(MUTTER MUSEUM,
PHILADELPHIA.)

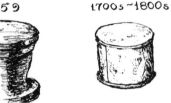

1780   1780

BLOWN GLASS   BLOWN GLASS
(BRAMBILLA~ INSTRUMENTARIUM.
CHIRURGICUM. VIENNESE. 1780.)

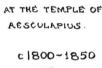

c1800~1850

PRESSED HORN
(MUTTER MUSEUM
PHILADELPHIA.)

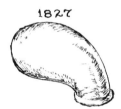

1827

"GLASS LEECH"

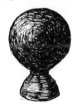
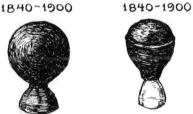

1840~1900

RUBBER
DR. FOX'S
(DAVIS +APPEL~BLOODLETTING INSTRUMENTS)

1840-1900

RUBBER, GLASS CUP
TIEMANN & CO. N.Y. 1889

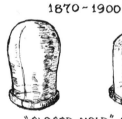

1870~1900

"CLOSED MOLD" GLASS
WITH MOLD SEAMS ON
BODY AND RIM.

Flint glass cups were by far the most popular from the seventeenth through the nineteenth centuries. Pontil marks were no longer found on glassware after the 1850s. These were round scars left after breaking of the pontil~ an iron rod that was attached to the glass base until the neck and rim could be finished. Thereafter, the cups were shaped in molds and not free-blown. A tell-tail mold seam could be seen on the body. The thick rim (thick enough to prevent injury to the skin when under vacuum) was applied between 1840~1880 as a "laid-on-ring" of molten glass. By 1870 the lip ring was part of the mold and the seam continued over it as well. Glass cups were often sold in sets of three or six glasses.

Cupping was also recommended as a counter-irritant, much as irritating poultices and hot caudery irons were used to blister the skin. By producing a new site of inflammation, the blood was sidetracked from

diseased engorged areas.
Inflamed joints, chest symptoms
such as coughing or breathlessness,
headaches, sore throat, cramps, lunacy,
convulsions, and a host of other bodily
miseries were fair game for the
business of cupping.

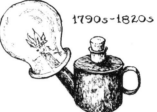

1851-1915 BAUNCHEIDT'S LEBENSWECKER

"LEBENSWECKER"
IS GERMAN FOR "LIFE
AWAKENER." THE HOLLOW
EBONY TUBE CONTAINED A HANDLE
WITH COILED SPRING ATTACHED. WHEN PUSHED, THE 30
SHARP NEEDLES PUNCTURED THE SKIN. THIS COUNTER-
IRRITANT WOULD "AWAKEN" ANYONE! (KNY SCHEERER 1915)

CUPPING BY VACUUM ~
a choice of either heating the inner cup or sucking out the air.

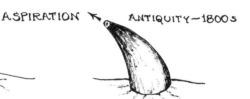

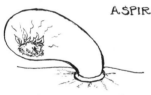

-HEAT- TO 1800+

A WAD OF BURNING
HEMP OR FLAX WAS PLACED IN
THE CUP WITH THE RIM IN CONTACT
WITH THE SKIN. ALTHOUGH WIDELY
USED, THE PATIENT MIGHT BE
SCORCHED. THERE WERE BETTER WAYS.

1708

DIONIS USED SMALL
CANDLES ON A CARD
TO PROTECT THE SKIN
WHILE EXHAUSTING
THE AIR.

1790s-1820s

THE TIN "TEAPOT"
LAMP FILLED WITH
ALCOHOL, HEATED THE
CUP WITH ITS COTTON
WICK JUST BEFORE
PLACEMENT ON THE SKIN.

1820~1900

CUPPING TORCH-
A BEVELED TUBE
STUFFED WITH
COTTON WAS DIPPED
IN ALCOHOL AND LIT.
BEST HEAT SOURCE YET.

1820

FOX'S "GLASS LEECH"
COULD BURN THE LINT
INSIDE THE GLASS WITH-
OUT SINGEING.

ASPIRATION → ANTIQUITY-1800s

THE COW'S HORN WAS
THE COMMON MAN'S CUPPER.
AFTER AIR WAS SUCKED BY
MOUTH THROUGH A HOLE
BORED DOWN THE TIP, IT WAS
THEN PLUGGED WITH WAX.

1100s~1800s

CERAMIC SPOUTED
CUPPING GLASS.
PERSIAN.
(DAVIS + APPEL - BLOOD-
LETTING INSTRUMENTS.)

1840~1900

GLASS CUP WITH
VULCANIZED RUBBER
BULB REVOLUTIONIZED
CUPPING. LIGHT AND
INEXPENSIVE. A SQUEEZE
GAVE INSTANT VACUUM.

DRY VS. WET CUPPING

Dry cupping brought congestion to a local body surface without injury to
the skin. Blood was mobilized and shifted, but not removed. This further step
toward good health was a job for the lancet. A series of parallel incisions
would be made after a sponge with hot water had dilated the capillaries. This
painful, bloody procedure could easily make the patient forget his original complaints.
Cupping followed to draw the blood from the tiny surface vessels more freely.
This was wet cupping. It was the usual practice to
draw up from three to five ounces of excess   c1680
blood in each glass applied.

THE SCARIFICATOR   A more merciful
device, the scarificator, made its first slashes
in the early 1700s. Multiple blades
shot out at the flick of the release   BRASS 2 BLADED
lever, creating an instantaneous   SCARIFICATOR SIMILAR
series of parallel cuts. Until the   TO BENNION-ANT. MED. INST.

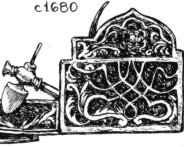

early 1800s these blades were pointed. Thereafter, the multiple blades were larger and curved to give a cleaner series of cuts. Twelve blades were usual, but others held six to twenty blades.

The earlier boxes were square, and the German models remained so through the 1800s. By 1790, the octagonal scarificator was favored by the English and Americans. Round boxes, often French in origin, were in use between 1850 to 1900. Some instruments were sold after 1900, but by then the practice had quietly passed on to a well-deserved death.

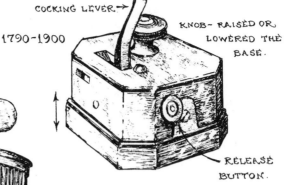

COCKING LEVER →

1790-1900

KNOB - RAISED OR LOWERED THE BASE.

1850~1900

COCKING LEVER

RELEASE BUTTON.

RELEASE BUTTON.

OCTAGONAL SCARIFICATOR WITH HOUSING OF BRASS. DEPTH OF THE 13 BLADES WAS ADJUSTED BY RAISING OR LOWERING THE BASE.

ROUND SCARIFICATOR OF WHITE ALLOY METAL. TURNING BASE REGULATES THE DEPTH OF THE 6 BLADES.

SYRINGE ~ CUP COMBINATIONS

c 1800~1900

c 1850~1900

Since the late 1700s, the sophisticated wet cupping circles welcomed an ongoing parade of aspirating syringes that could be screwed on to a glass cup fitting. Sucking out the air from a cup with one's mouth had none of the niceties of a syringe~cup set. In a velvet lined mahogany case one could find an impressive brass syringe, graduated cupping glasses with brass stopcocks and a brass scarificator. Professional and proper, indeed. Despite the popularity of such combinations, the profes~ sional cupper found the sticky valves and stopcocks, as well as the bother of attaching and removing the syringe, not at all to their liking.

THE TUBE ATTACHMENT GAVE PLAY SO THAT THE CUP REMAINED SECURE ON THE SKIN.

THE MECHANICAL (ARTIFICIAL) LEECH

The next step was to mimic that very successful creature, the leech. The first half of the 1800s had some false starts, each as ingenious as it was impractical.

By the middle of the century a French inventor, Charles Heurteloup produced his two piece artificial leech. First, a scarifier was rotated by pulling a cord. Then, a syringe was positioned over the puncture and the screw created suction as the plunger rose. The device was quite popular ~ especially for bleeding

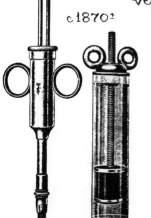

c 1870±

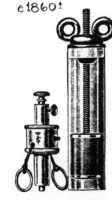

c 1860±

c 1870±

LUER'S CUTTER AND ARTIFICIAL LEECH.

HEURTELOUP'S CUTTER AND ARTIFICIAL LEECH.

ILLUSTRATIONS FROM KNY SCHEERER CATALOGUE 1915~ STILL ADVERTIZING BLOODLETTERS AT THIS LATE DATE !

BACON'S SPRING-LOADED SCARIFIER AND CUPPING CUP.

the temples as a treatment for eye afflictions.

Dr. Reese's "Uterine Leech," in use by 1876, went one step further. This all-in-one instrument contained a spear lancet that moved freely through the plunger. After the puncture, the lancet was withdrawn by a coiled spring and the blood could be suctioned immediately. The long narrow cylinder made the chore of cupping the cervix considerably easier. It was as close to the functions of the leech as any, but as timely as last week's newspaper. Bleeding was becoming little more than a regretable memory.

REECE'S "UTERINE LEECH. (KNY SCHEERER 1915)

LEECHES nature's answer to the mania for letting blood.

Not all leeches from the class Hirudinea and phylum Annelida could qualify for local blood depletion. Most scavenged from dead animal matter or small cold-blooded snails and shellfish. About 100 B.C., Syrian physicians were putting a true medicinal leech (Hirudo medicinalis) to work drawing bad blood from their patients. This species lived out its six years of life in the stagnant shallow fresh waters of Europe. From two to three inches long, it was distinguished by the olive green skin that was ornamented with four yellow longitudinal lines, the center two being interrupted with black.

THE MEDICINAL LEECH.

The Greeks and Romans carried on the practice, and by the Middle Ages, leeching was a way of life for both physicians and barbers. In fact, the word leech comes from the medieval English word "leche" meaning "physician."

Northern American colonists found a bonanza of another medical species in their own sluggish streams and ponds, the Macrobdella decora. These leeches were an impressive lot, sometimes growing up to nine inches in length. With their green, orange and black markings made them handsome ~ at least in the eyes of their fellows. Unfortunately (or fortunately) they were far less hungry than their European cousins. It took six American leeches to draw an ounce of blood, whereas a single European leech (or Swedish leech as it was sometimes called) could draw the same amount without any help. Therefore most physicians on this side of the Atlantic preferred to import whenever possible.

The leech secures itself (since a leech is both male and female and a pair fertilize each other's eggs, "it" it must be) with a large suction cup at one end. At the other end is a smaller suction cup, in the center of which are three sharp teeth that make a triangular puncture. Once made, it injects an anticoagulant, hirudin, to produce a clot-free meal.

A leech was useful for removing blood from confined spaces such as the larynx, trachea, around the eyes, the rectum, and the vagina. By smearing the skin with a dab of blood or a little sugar and water, it could be encouraged to bite at a selected site. When placed in a small cup next to the inflammation or hematoma (such as a "black eye," the worm would crawl out and attach itself. To prevent any wandering within a bodily cavity, leech tubes directed their aim while confining it to the bleeding

1863

A GLASS FUNNEL, OPEN AT BOTH ENDS, DIRECTED THE LEECH TO SPECIFIC SITES FOR DRAINING HEMATOMAS.
(SMITH-PRINCIPLES, PRACTICE OF SURGERY 1863)

area. It would drop off when full and have no desire for another feeding for several months.

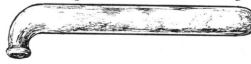

LEECH TUBES.

LEECH CONTAINERS

Leeches were kept in holding jars that held water - and it must be frequently changed. A blown glass bowl, not unlike those holding fish, was popular in America. Since leeches could inch themselves along on a dry surface much like their worm relatives, a widely turned lip was needed. A piece of gauze could then be placed over the mouth of the bowl and tied below the lip. The escape route was then secured, and at the same time allowed free passage of air. The French version was similar, except that the bowl perched on a glass pedestal and disc-like base.

Better known were the ceramic jars and urn-shaped containers that might range from a plain cylinder to a heavily embellished piece. In any event, each must have a lid with multiple air holes. Some recent reproductions can confuse identification of the old, but can be quickly discounted if the lid holes are absent. The English excelled at the very ornate ceramic pieces, although they and the Germans made plain cylindrical back room jars for less spectacular leech storage.

LEECH CARRIER OF PEWTER, DRAWN FULL SCALE. 19TH CENTURY. (WELLCOME MUSEUM, LONDON)

LATE 18TH TO MID-19TH CENTURY.

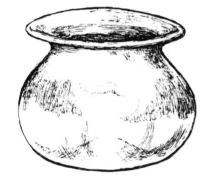

AMERICAN BLOWN GLASS BOWL - NOT TO BE CONFUSED WITH THE THICK LIPPED CUPPING GLASSES. A SET WOULD INCLUDE HEIGHTS OF $2\frac{1}{4}"$, $2\frac{3}{4}"$, $4"$, $5\frac{1}{2}"$, $7"$ AND $9\frac{1}{4}"$ NOTE THE EXTENDED LIP FOR TYING.

c.1890s

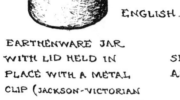

EARTHENWARE JAR WITH LID HELD IN PLACE WITH A METAL CLIP (JACKSON-VICTORIAN CHEMIST AND DRUGGIST)

c.1810

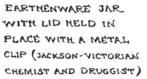

ENGLISH.

PLATED TRAVELLING LEECH BOX $\frac{1}{2}$ SIZE. CARRIED LEECHES ON HOUSE CALLS AS WITH THE LEECH CARRIER. (WELLCOME MUSEUM, LONDON)

c.1830

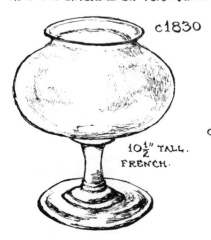

$10\frac{1}{2}"$ TALL. FRENCH.

c.1900

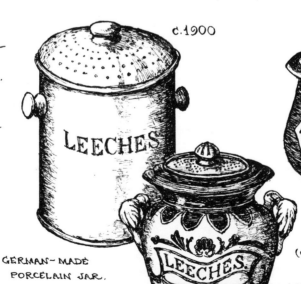

GERMAN-MADE PORCELAIN JAR.

c.1830-40

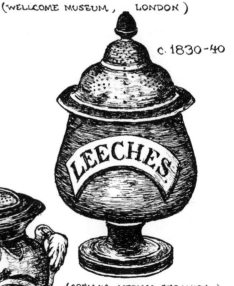

(CRELLIN-MEDICAL CERAMICS...)

1842~1853 (CRELLIN-MEDICAL CERAMICS IN THE WELLCOME INSTITUTE, LONDON)

VACCINATION LANCETS

To our early colonists, the dreaded smallpox must have seemed the devil's own curse. The Reverend Dr. Mather, no stranger to combat with the forces of evil, first suggested inoculation of Americans as prophylaxis. His close friend, Dr. Zabdiel Boylston, thought on the idea, and on June 27, 1721 inoculated his thirteen year old son and two black servants. His experiment came just two months after being tried in England, and it proved an unqualified success.

Dr. Boylston carried his crusade to 247 others that year and into early 1722. An additional 39 Americans were treated by other doctors. Only 6 died of the procedure, and it was likely that several of those had contracted the disease before inoculation. During that same period, 5754 had caught the disease in the "natural" way, and of these, 844 died. Many of the others were disfigured for life.

Dr. Boylston's method was to "Take your Medicine or Pus from the ripe pustule of the Small Pox of the distinct kind, either from those in the natural way or from the inoculated sort, provided the person be other-wise healthy and the matter good. My way of taking it is thus: Take a fine cut, sharp toothpick (which will not put the person in any fear, as a Lancet will do many), and open the Pock on one side, and press the Boil, and scoop the matter on your quill, and so on."

1798 was the year for one of medicine's great milestones. Dr. Edward Jenner of England discovered the cowpox virus vaccination to be a smallpox preventative without the possible complications from a pox pustule. A profes-sor of medicine at Harvard, Dr. Benjamin Waterhouse, had some of the vaccine sent to him two years later. His first patients were his four children, and they remained free of the disease after repeated exposure.

By the 1970s, smallpox was so well controlled that vaccination was only given to those in or visiting endemic areas.

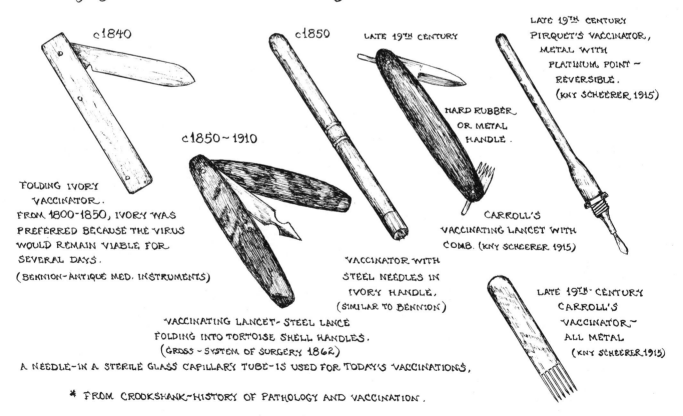

c1840

c1850

LATE 19TH CENTURY

LATE 19TH CENTURY PIRQUET'S VACCINATOR, METAL WITH PLATINUM POINT ~ REVERSIBLE. (KNY SCHEERER 1915)

c1850~1910

HARD RUBBER OR METAL HANDLE.

FOLDING IVORY VACCINATOR. FROM 1800-1850, IVORY WAS PREFERRED BECAUSE THE VIRUS WOULD REMAIN VIABLE FOR SEVERAL DAYS. (BENNION-ANTIQUE MED. INSTRUMENTS)

CARROLL'S VACCINATING LANCET WITH COMB. (KNY SCHEERER 1915)

VACCINATOR WITH STEEL NEEDLES IN IVORY HANDLE. (SIMILAR TO BENNION)

VACCINATING LANCET-STEEL LANCE FOLDING INTO TORTOISE SHELL HANDLES. (GROSS - SYSTEM OF SURGERY 1862)

LATE 19TH CENTURY CARROLL'S VACCINATOR ~ ALL METAL (KNY SCHEERER 1915)

A NEEDLE~IN A STERILE GLASS CAPILLARY TUBE-IS USED FOR TODAY'S VACCINATIONS.

* FROM CROOKSHANK~HISTORY OF PATHOLOGY AND VACCINATION.

AMPUTATION INSTRUMENTS

Loose a limb and save a life ~ that was the goal in the pre-Lister days of sterilization when a wound might be followed by a galloping infection. Some four hundred years ago the French army surgeon, Ambrose Paré, called it "signs of a perfect Necrosis or Mortification." Only amputation could prevent certain death from putrification that would "creepe and spread over the rest of the body." In the seventeenth century, the "father of English surgery," Richard Wiseman recommended primary amputations (an operation before the onset of fever).

Yet before Paré (1509~1590), amputation was hardly a guarantee that the mysterious and deadly necrosis could be controlled. In the days when barbers and surgeons were much the same, the stump was often brutalized with boiling oil and roasted with red-hot caudery irons to control post-surgery bleeding. A fatal fever could be the end result.

Paré's great contribution was to re-introduce the old Greek and Roman use of ligatures for tying off the cut vessels. The stump was then covered with clean bandages. The number of amputation complications dropped dramatically, and Paré's place in surgical history was assured.

THE TOURNIQUET   Paré compressed the arteries above the amputation site by tying a simple ligature. Fabriz von Hilden (1560~1634) introduced another simple sort of tourniquet. A handle of wood was twisted under the strap that encircled the limb. In 1718, Jean Louis Petit (1674~1750) popularized his screw tourniquet ~ the standard means of working in a bloodless field until the early 1900s. As with its predecessors, compression of the nerves as well, gave some numbing of the pain to a small degree.

Many other compressing devices, all inferior, were devised. The "Field Tourniquet" was a simple strap and buckle that was some-times given to soldiers in time of war for emergency first aid. Unless firmly

Serratum.

HANS GERSDORFF'S FELDTBUCH DER WUNDARTZNEY, 1540. THIS FIRST WOODCUT OF AN AMPUTATION SHOWED TOURNIQUET BANDAGES CHECKING HEMORRHAGE AS THE SAW SEVERED THE BONES. RATHER THAN USE CAUDERY, THE SURGEON USED STYPTICS OF LIME, VITRIOL, ALUM, ALOES AND NUTGALLS. THE STUMP WAS THEN COVERED WITH THE BLADDER FROM AN OX OR HOG.

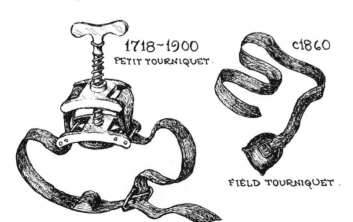

1718~1900
PETIT TOURNIQUET.

c1860

FIELD TOURNIQUET.

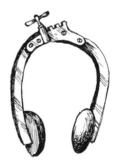

SIGNORONI'S HORSE-SHOE TOURNIQUET.

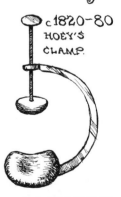

c1820~80
HOEY'S CLAMP.

SIMILAR CLAMPS WERE IN USE SINCE THE MID-1700s.

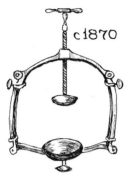

c 1870

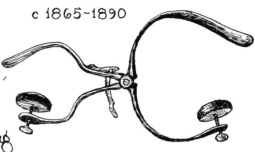

c 1865~1890

applied, they did more harm than good by cutting off venous flow without stopping the arterial hemorrhage. Also there were the Signoroni's, and Skey's tourniquets, Hoey's clamp and Gross's arterial compressor that seemed better suited for compression of aneurysms and temporary bleeding control than for amputations. Touted for bloodless

SKEY'S TOURNIQUET

GROSS'S ARTERIAL COMPRESSOR

surgery, Esmarch's India rubber roller bandage was applied c1860~1920. Although it squeezed the vessels dry, there was an annoying amount of oozing after being removed following amputation. It fell by the wayside.

AMPUTATION KNIVES

Although the common circular gillotine method was practiced by most Roman surgeons, some of the more enlightened preferred the flap amputation. Two oblique slices were made down to the bone and the soft tissues then retracted. The bone was sawed, the vessels tied and the flaps joined without the usual skin undercutting and bone stripping of the circular cut. Time saved meant less pain, and heaven knows there was more than enough of that without anesthesia. The flaps, with less trauma and contamination, healed nicely and was well cushioned for the artificial limb that would follow. A straight knife was used to divide the tissue.

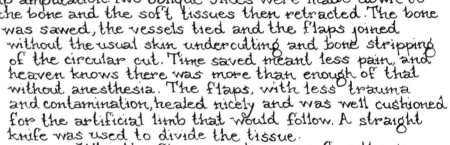

THE FLAP AMPUTATION

CUT WEDGE OF TWO HALF CIRCLES.

CROSS-SECTION-COMPLETED.

(FROM NATHAN SMITH, M.D.- MEMOIRS 1831 U.S.A.)

Why the flap operation was forgotten in the medieval centuries - appropriately called the dark ages - remains a head-scratcher. Dr. Loudham, an Oxford surgeon, did his best to re-introduce the flap amputation in 1679 but stirred up little enthusiasm. Yet it WAS being done. Dr. Knyveton* recalled his apprenticeship days in 1751. An attorney's clerk had fallen and suffered a compound fracture of the lower leg. "The clerk in great pain and the wound discharging through part of his black stocking having been caught by the bone and drawn into the wound. The wound about the exit of the bone very foul the flesh about swollen and the skin hard and shiny to half-way up the shin; so that the Doctor did resolve to remove the leg at the knee. The clerk was taken from his bed in Great Lowness.... Then the clerk being bound his leg was held out firmly by the aforesaid servant who wedged it against his belly and Dr. Urqueham [of London] with a sharp knife cuts a half-circle from below the Tubercle of the Tibia to the middle of the joint behind and repeats same on the opposing side and I pull these flaps back and get soaked with blood from the great arteries at which the Doctor laughs... then he ligates the vessels with cords and sews up the two flaps leaving the ends of the ligature cords hanging from the wound. The Doctor a very quick man and the leg off in four minutes, though due to my clumsiness another minute or two elapsed before the wound was secured. I have heard and can believe that when he Amputates with another cunning and experienced surgeon only two or three minutes elapse before it is complete. And so the clerk was removed in all Peace he having fainted from the Vehemence of His Emotions at the cutting of the second flap and I for one very thankful, for his screams at the first nigh deafened me."

The circular amputation had little to recommend it. A curved-bladed

* KNYVETON'S THE DIARY OF A SURGEON 1752.

124

THE CIRCULAR AMPUTATION AS CARRIED OUT IN THE AMERICAN REVOLUTION PERIOD.

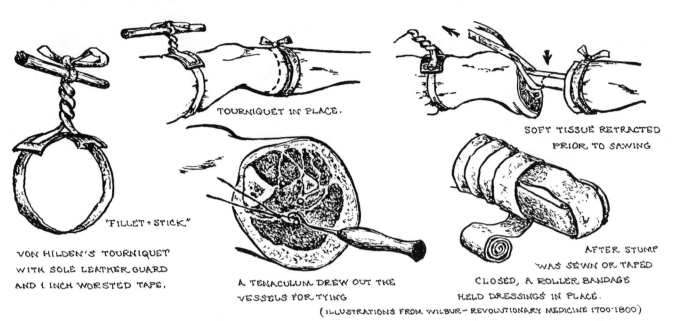

TOURNIQUET IN PLACE.

SOFT TISSUE RETRACTED
PRIOR TO SAWING

"FILLET + STICK"

VON HILDEN'S TOURNIQUET
WITH SOLE LEATHER GUARD
AND 1 INCH WORSTED TAPE.

A TENACULUM DREW OUT THE
VESSELS FOR TYING

AFTER STUMP
WAS SEWN OR TAPED
CLOSED, A ROLLER BANDAGE
HELD DRESSINGS IN PLACE.

(ILLUSTRATIONS FROM WILBUR - REVOLUTIONARY MEDICINE 1700-1800)

knife, much like a sickle, was used to sweep around the skin. After being encircled, the skin was freed from the muscles with a scalpel and drawn back. The muscles were cut in the same way above the previous incision. The muscles were retracted in turn after being separated from the bone. After the bone was sawed, the arteries were tied and the soft parts pulled together and secured. The limb, but not the duration of pain, was shortened appreciably by the circular amputation method. Our Revolutionary War soldiers continued to loose their arms in the same old circular amputation way. Only the knife blade was changing, for it was becoming much less curved or was entirely straight.

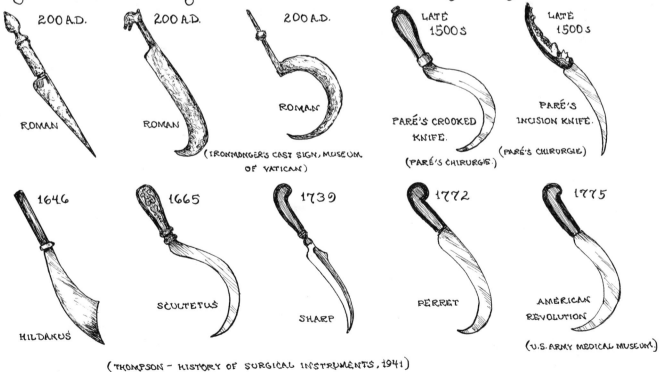

200 A.D. — ROMAN

200 A.D. — ROMAN

200 A.D. — ROMAN
(IRONMONGER'S CAST SIGN, MUSEUM
OF VATICAN)

LATE 1500s — PARÉ'S CROOKED KNIFE.
(PARÉ'S CHIRURGIE.)

LATE 1500s — PARÉ'S INCISION KNIFE.
(PARÉ'S CHIRURGIE)

1646 — HILDANUS

1665 — SCULTETUS

1739 — SHARP

1772 — PERRET

1775 — AMERICAN REVOLUTION
(U.S. ARMY MEDICAL MUSEUM.)

(THOMPSON - HISTORY OF SURGICAL INSTRUMENTS, 1941)

THE CRESCENT~SHAPED BLADES CONTINUED THROUGHOUT THE FIRST HALF OF THE 18TH CENTURY. BETWEEN 1760~1775 THE CURVED BLADE VARIED IN SHAPE, AND BY 1775 IT BECAME NEARLY STRAIGHT. MOST HANDLES IN THE 18TH CENTURY WERE OF LIGNUM VITAE OR EBONY AND WERE OCTAGONALLY SHAPED ON CROSS SECTION WITH THE TERMINAL END CURVING INWARD OR OUTWARD.

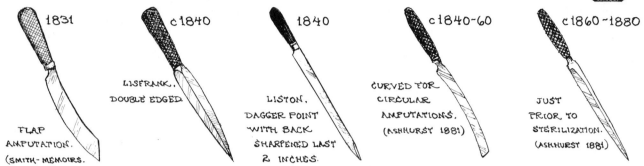

1831
FLAP AMPUTATION.
(SMITH- MEMOIRS. USA. 1831)

c1840
LISFRANK. DOUBLE EDGED

1840
LISTON. DAGGER POINT WITH BACK SHARPENED LAST 2 INCHES.

c1840-60
CURVED FOR CIRCULAR AMPUTATIONS. (ASHHURST 1881)

c1860~1880
JUST PRIOR TO STERILIZATION. (ASHHURST 1881)

It took the energies and reputations of Robert Liston and James Syme of England to bring back the old flap amputations. The six-foot tall Liston, with large and powerful hands to match, could slice out a wedge-shaped stump of soft tissue with two strokes of his straight foot-long blade. In just three minutes the ordeal was over. His speed and skill were a guarantee of a useful stump. Both he and Symes published their favorable flap results in England in 1824. Speed was essential until the mid-1800s. Then, chloroform and ether permitted a more careful and considered approach ~ just in time for the Civil War carnage.

By 1870, many of the straight amputation blades were double-edged for about an inch from the point. They were used for both the flap and the circular amputations. As for size, Liston insisted that "The form and size of the instruments ought always be in proportion to the extent of the proposed excision as regards to both their length and depth. Nothing can possibly be imagined more abominably cruel, for instance, than the attempt (which has to my knowledge been repeatedly made and which I have in fact witnessed) to remove the lower extremity of a full-grown person with a common scalpel or dissecting knife." As a rule of thumb, the knife length should be about 1½ times the diameter of the limb, and its width from $\frac{3}{8}$ to $\frac{3}{4}$ of an inch. For example, a cutting edge of 8 or 9 inches would be used on the thigh, and a 6 to 7 inch blade for smaller limbs.

Nineteenth century handles were of ebony or ivory and were checkered for a firm grip. Liston was much in the minority with his smooth and polished handles. He felt checkered grasps did not give a delicacy of touch and only for those who were "...more afraid of loosing hold of the instrument in a fit of agitation and panic..." And smooth handles did become standard when the importance of aseptic surgery in 1860 became known. Wood or ivory checkered handles were favorite hiding places for bacteria, and sterilization called for smooth metal handles. Old ways die hard, and late nineteenth century catalogues still advertized the ebony handles.

Briefly, there were smaller amputation knives used for specialized tasks.

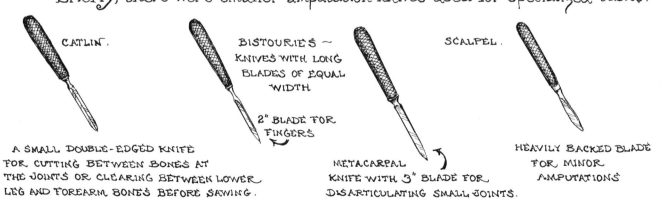

CATLIN.
A SMALL DOUBLE-EDGED KNIFE FOR CUTTING BETWEEN BONES AT THE JOINTS OR CLEARING BETWEEN LOWER LEG AND FOREARM BONES BEFORE SAWING.

BISTOURIES ~ KNIVES WITH LONG BLADES OF EQUAL WIDTH
2" BLADE FOR FINGERS

METACARPAL KNIFE WITH 3" BLADE FOR DISARTICULATING SMALL JOINTS.

SCALPEL.
HEAVILY BACKED BLADE FOR MINOR AMPUTATIONS

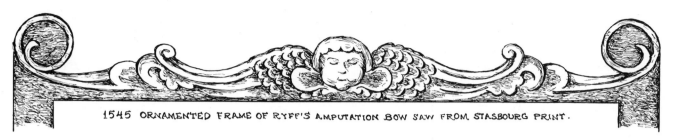

1545 ORNAMENTED FRAME OF RYFF'S AMPUTATION BOW SAW FROM STASBOURG PRINT.

AMPUTATION SAWS

AMPUTATION SAWS ~ The bone of the human limb was sawed much like that of a tree limb. The bone covering (periosteum-the bone growth layer) was first cut with a scalpel close to the retracted muscles. With the saw in this guideline, the blade was drawn toward the operator until a track was deep enough for to-and-fro cuts. When nearly sawed through, the blade was angled to prevent an irregular break. Meanwhile, the limb was supported only enough to prevent the saw from binding.

BEFORE 3300 B.C.

The earliest known saw was used by the Egyptians some four thousand years ago. The ancient Greeks made the dividing of bone easier with copper blades, followed by those of the more durable bronze.

EGYPTIAN SAW WITH FLINT BLADES IN WOODEN HAFT (BRITISH MUSEUM.)

The Romans, about 200 B.C., introduced the prototypes for the coming centuries. Their most popular blade was the tenon style that resembled the ordinary carpenter's saw. The bow saw or frame pattern was also in evidence and looked like today's hacksaw. A glance at the comparative anatomy of these and the later versions will show how little some medical instruments have changed. The blades were of sturdy iron or steel.

BEFORE 200 B.C.
ROMAN TENON BROAD-BLADED SAW.
(BRITISH MUSEUM.)

c 200 B.C.
ROMAN BOW SAW FROM A STONE RELIEF IN THE MUSEC DU CAPITOLE, ROME.
STEEL BLADE.

By the 1500s, surgical saws had become works of art. Usually of a heavy bow construction, the out-sized frame was embellished with fine decorations. The lathe-turned or carved handles were of wood, bone, or ivory. To keep the blade tight, a screw device was pioneered by Walter Hermann Ryff about 1545. By the mid-1600s, Scultetus used the idea as a thumbscrew that passed through the handle.

c 1545

BOW ~

RYFF'S SURGICAL SAW WITH AN END SCREW FOR TIGHTENING THE BLADE.
(THOMPSON - HIST. EVOLUTION SURG. INST.)

MID -1600s

BOW ~

SCULTETUS ~ HANDLE WITH TIGHTENING SCREW.
(THOMPSON)

In the late 1700s, the tenon blade was making a gradual comeback. It was certainly a sturdier instrument than the bow or frame saw, and was further reinforced by a steel spine. This was a period of innovations. One of the most interesting was a guarded blade that could cut the bone without injury to the surrounding muscle.

Certainly the most enduring amputation saw concept from the eighteenth century was the chain saw. With it, bones that were nearly surrounded by soft tissue could be handily divided. A curved needle was tied to the free end of the chain links and then carried under the bone with the cutting edges

18TH CENTURY

GUARDED AMPUTATION SAW WITH THUMB SCREWS FOR SETTING THE WIDTH OF THE GUARD
(THOMPSON - HISTORY + EVOLUTION OF SURGICAL INSTRUMENTS)

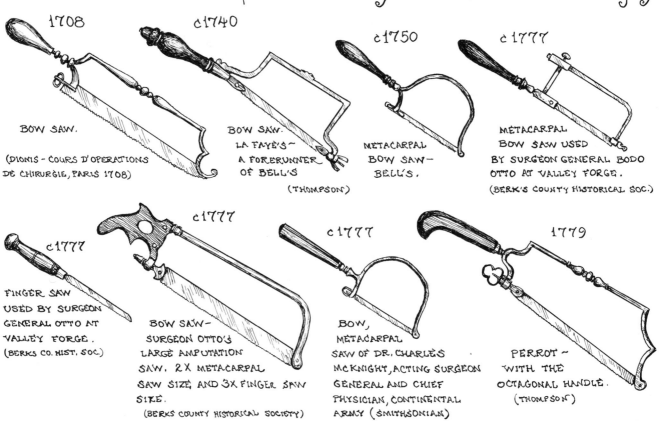

c1791

CHAIN SAW.

(BRYANT - OPERATIVE SURGERY 1902)

upward. When the "T" handle was substituted for the needle, the instrument could be drawn from side to side at a forty-five degree angle. A later improvement was the Gigli-Haertel saw with chain links that cut in any position. The Gigli was less expensive, easily cleaned and was less apt to bind. It is in use for today's amputations.

During the eighteenth century, handles had also undergone changes. The bow saw turned handles gave way in the early 1770s to smooth handles that were hexagonal on cross-section. Twenty years later, checkered grooves became popular and assured the surgeon of a firmer grip. This cross-hatching continued until the 1870~1880s when sterilization of surgical instruments was generally appreciated. Thereafter, saws were much less visually appealing and were one piece of steel, the frame nickle-plated and perfectly smooth to prevent rust and without crevices where bacteria could set up housekeeping. Each could be boiled and then placed in the early carbolic solutions without injury.

1708

BOW SAW.

(DIONIS - COURS D'OPERATIONS DE CHIRURGIE, PARIS 1708)

c1740

BOW SAW. LA FAYE'S ~ A FORERUNNER OF BELL'S

(THOMPSON)

c1750

METACARPAL BOW SAW ~ BELL'S.

c1777

METACARPAL BOW SAW USED BY SURGEON GENERAL BODO OTTO AT VALLEY FORGE.

(BERK'S COUNTY HISTORICAL SOC.)

c1777

FINGER SAW USED BY SURGEON GENERAL OTTO AT VALLEY FORGE.

(BERKS CO. HIST. SOC.)

c1777

BOW SAW ~ SURGEON OTTO'S LARGE AMPUTATION SAW. 2 X METACARPAL SAW SIZE AND 3X FINGER SAW SIZE.

(BERKS COUNTY HISTORICAL SOCIETY)

c1777

BOW, METACARPAL SAW OF DR. CHARLES McKNIGHT, ACTING SURGEON GENERAL AND CHIEF PHYSICIAN, CONTINENTAL ARMY (SMITHSONIAN)

1779

PERROT ~ WITH THE OCTAGONAL HANDLE.

(THOMPSON)

The nineteenth century surgeons were finding the tenon saw a cut above the time-honored bow saw. As for handle form, small saws generally had grips that resembled those of a table knife. Larger saws carried either pistol handles with or without finger holes or those like fancy carpenters' saws.

The bow saw was not entirely forgotten. Richard Butcher gave his name, with its unfortunate connotation, to a modified version. Butcher recommended its use for curving the amputated bone and for its ease in sawing under the flaps without injury to the surrounding muscle or catching on the retractor.

All in all, the concept of the bow saw, chain saw and tenon saw have changed but little throughout the twentieth century.

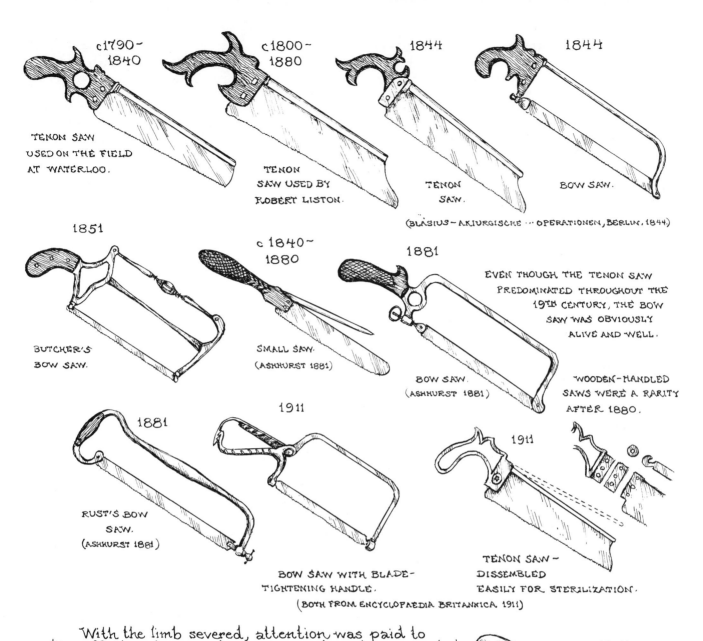

c1790–1840
TENON SAW
USED ON THE FIELD
AT WATERLOO.

c1800–1880
TENON
SAW USED BY
ROBERT LISTON.

1844
TENON
SAW.

1844
BOW SAW.
(BLASIUS – AKIURGISCHE ··· OPERATIONEN, BERLIN, 1844)

1851
BUTCHER'S
BOW SAW.

c1840–1880
SMALL SAW.
(ASHHURST 1881)

1881
BOW SAW.
(ASHHURST 1881)

EVEN THOUGH THE TENON SAW
PREDOMINATED THROUGHOUT THE
19ᵀᴴ CENTURY, THE BOW
SAW WAS OBVIOUSLY
ALIVE AND WELL.

WOODEN–HANDLED
SAWS WERE A RARITY
AFTER 1880.

1881
RUST'S BOW
SAW.
(ASHHURST 1881)

1911
BOW SAW WITH BLADE–
TIGHTENING HANDLE.
(BOTH FROM ENCYCLOPAEDIA BRITANNICA 1911)

1911
TENON SAW –
DISSEMBLED
EASILY FOR STERILIZATION.

1973
MODERN
BOW SAW WITH
SOLID OR LOOP
HANDLE.
(MILEX INSTRUMENT CO. 1973)

With the limb severed, attention was paid to sealing off the stump arteries. As mentioned, open-ended bodily plumbing was seared with a red-hot iron prior to Paré. Through his efforts, the famous French surgeon popularized the tying off of vessels as noted in the "Artery Forceps" section. Ligatures were of waxed flax or silk threads, and even after the Civil War were well contaminated by surgeons who found their buttonhole a handy ligature holder. Because of the infection that inevitably followed, the stump was only partially sutured. The ligatures were left long and left hanging from one end of the wound. From day to day, they were gently tugged until they came away.

Lister insisted on making these ligatures aseptic by boiling, then set about developing an absorbable ligature. At long last, the closure of the stump could be completed without the danger of infection around each tie.

18ᵀᴴ CENTURY CAUDERY IRON.

TREPANNING AND TREPHINING

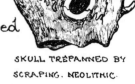

SKULL TREPANNED BY
SCRAPING. NEOLITHIC.
(MEMOIRES ··· DE BAYE)

Unconcious and barely alive, the ancient Peruvian warrior was carried from the field of battle with a portion of his skull indented by an enemy war club. Assistants held the unfortunate's arms and legs to the ground while the surgeon anchored the head firmly between his knees. Over the depressed fracture, the scalp was incised with a chipped stone knife. With a hafted stone drill, a circle of holes were bored around the fracture lines, the bony bridges between them sawed or scraped, and the disc pried free. Less often, two parallel grooves were sawed with the chipped knife or copper blade at right angles to two like grooves. The bases of the bony splinters could then be removed. Occasionally the fracture site was simply scraped until the tough, fibrous brain covering (dura mater) was in sight.

BLADE
PROBABLY
WAS HAFTED.

It was a ticklish bit of surgery, for a sudden penetration of the sharp blade into the substance of the brain could send the warrior to his happy hunting ground. To forestall such a disaster, the blade was beveled to an increased thickness away from the cutting edge.

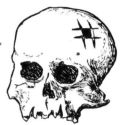

SKULL TREPANNED BY
CUTTING A SQUARE.
FROM VALLEY OF YUCARY,
PERU. (AMERICAN MUSEUM
OF NATURAL HISTORY LIBRARY)

In this business of trepanning, it should be mentioned that the entire fracture need not be removed. A small cut or bored hole, large enough to insert a prying instrument (elevator) might be all that was necessary to raise the depressed sections of bone to their normal position. Small unattached spicules would be excised. Then, to prevent brain herniation, a shell, animal bone or hammered piece of metal was fitted to replace any large trepanned piece of bone.

STONE AND
COPPER
TREPANNING
INSTRUMENTS
EXCAVATED IN PERU.

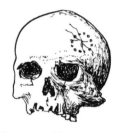

SKULL TREPANNED BY
DRILL HOLES, SCRAPING
BETWEEN, AND PRYING
FREE. (CONJECTURAL)

Impossible? Actually, the surgeons of those "primitive" tribes were highly skilled at their work. Between five and six percent of excavated Peruvian skulls showed just such an operation, and from the well-healed trepanned bones, it was clear that seventy-five percent survived the ordeal!

In addition to skull fractures, earlier Neolithic man trepanned for removing diseases of the skull and to release evil spirits causing such ailments as headaches and epilepsy.

By historic times, the basics of opening the skull remained the same, while the instruments for the purpose changed radically. One, the bone drill or "trepanon" made the boring of the circular pattern of skull holes considerably easier. The bony bridges between were scraped away with a lenticular or broken through with a sturdy scalpel. The other, the "terebra serrata," was a unique hollow cone of metal with saw teeth rimming its base. A center pin kept the saw from jumping its track while the handle was rotated between the palms.

THE "TREPANON"-AN
EARLY GREEK
BONE DRILL.

THE "TEREBRA
SERRATA," AN
EARLY GREEK CIRCULAR SAW.

THE TREPAN~ a frame or brace and bit much like a carpenter's drill.

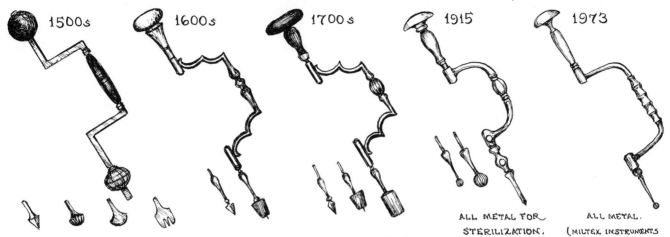

1500s   1600s   1700s   1915   1973

ALL METAL FOR
STERILIZATION.
(KNY-SCHEERER CO. 1915)

ALL METAL.
(MILTEX INSTRUMENTS
CO. 1973)

Andrea della Croce, a Venice teacher in the 1560s, combined the two concepts by using a brace and bit drill. His interchangeable bits were sharply pointed perforators or circular saws. Known as the trepan, it could be found in most of the surgicals sets from the sixteenth to the eighteenth centuries.

As for the center guide pin in the circular bit, the Romans had realized that once the round groove cut had been established, the pin must be removed. Failure to do so would mean puncture of the brain before the saw teeth had cut through the skull. A several step solution was described by Scultatus in his 1663 Armentarium Chirgicum. A male circular cutter, with its guide pin, first established the groove. The sawing of the skull disc was completed by substituting the pinless female bit.

By the mid-1500s, many of the saw drums were slightly flared instead of being cylindrical with straight sides. The slanted sides of the bored skull helped prevent a sudden penetration into the underlying brain.

The trepan served the surgeon long and well, but it had two disadvantages. Both hands were needed for the drilling, and there was a lack of delicacy when applying pressure with the instrument. A sudden breakthrough would endanger the brain tissue underneath.

THE TREPHINE (tree-FINE) solved both these problems. Fabricius (1537-1619) first described the "T" shaped skull drill with its three functional ends (tres fines). It was a multipurpose tool with one end of the lengthy handle grooved as a raspiratory for scraping and smoothing the trephined hole. Its other end was a smooth elevator for raising the skull disc and loose fractured spicules. The third end was, of course, the interchangeable perforator or circular saw bit.

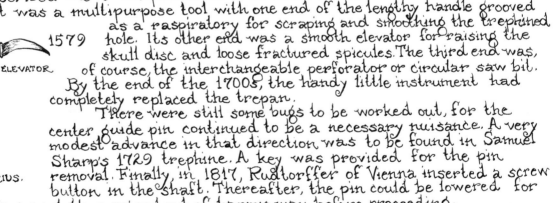

1579

RASPIRATORY   ELEVATOR

SAW BIT

TREPHINE~FABRICIUS.

By the end of the 1700s, the handy little instrument had completely replaced the trepan.

There were still some bugs to be worked out, for the center guide pin continued to be a necessary nuisance. A very modest advance in that direction was to be found in Samuel Sharp's 1729 trephine. A key was provided for the pin removal. Finally, in 1817, Rudtorffer of Vienna inserted a screw button in the shaft. Thereafter, the pin could be lowered for the initial sawing and then raised out of harm's way before proceeding.

Benjamin Bell's 1801 trephine featured three long gaps in the saw-toothed drum. The bone sawdust that collected was freed through the slots. Thereafter, the instrument was essentially unchanged. By the 1830s, the trephine was found useful for sawing out necrotic or diseased areas from the long bones of the extremities. By the late 1800s, it was replaced by a revival of the old bit and saw trepan.

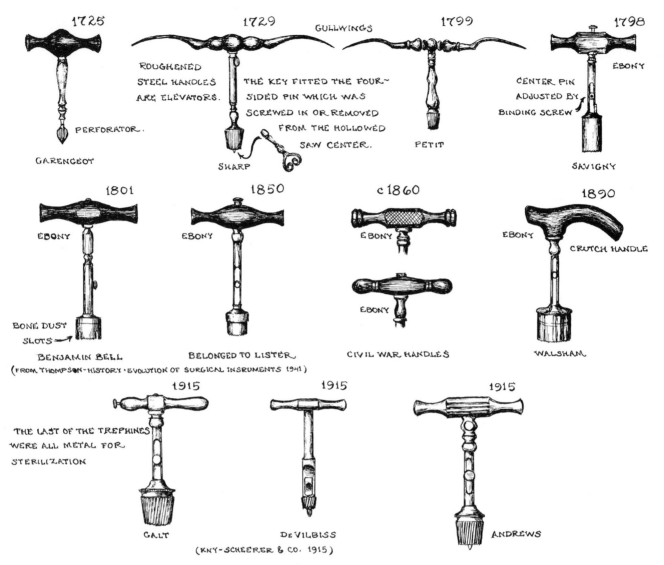

HEAD SAWS ~

It would be a rare trepanning or trephining set that did not include the following ~

As we have seen, the Peruvian Indians were doing creditable trepanning well over 4000 years ago. Their chipped stone blades were among the earliest known head saws for cutting a square hole or sawing between drilled skull holes. Although the Grecian modiolus was an efficient replacement for removing a bone disc rather than a square, there was want of a mini-saw to connect the perforator holes around more extensive skull fractures.

Not until the twelfth century did the Chirurgie of Albucasis describe just such a specialized saw with a nearly rounded blade. Although later head saws became more gently curved, the medieval surgeons seemed happy enough with the design. By the sixteenth century, it was realized that a combined straight and curved saw edges could produce a smoother trepanned opening. The two forms crafted as single or two-bladed head saws until the early eighteenth century. The rising popularity of the circular saw disc bit temporarily displaced the perforator and the head saw in the early eighteenth century.

By 1783, the small saw was back in the running, thanks to a revival by Cockell, a surgeon at Pontefract. His enthusiasm was catching, and William Hey, the senior surgeon at England's Leeds Infirmary, spent some twenty years experimenting with various head saw shapes and sizes. In his 1803 <u>Practical Observations on Surgery</u>, Hey reported that the efficient little saw could all but replace the trephine.

He went on to say "Dr. Cockell's saw has a semi-lunear edge, but the edge may be straight or of any degree of convexity which may be thought most useful. The straight-edged saw executes its task with great readiness, but the convex edge is necessary when the bone is to be sawed in a curvilinear direction. It is also useful when the thickness of that part of the cranium which is to be sawed through is very unequal."

As a result of Hey's research, the head saw in all its forms has since been generically called "Hey's saw."

1500s AND THEREAFTER

DOUBLE-BLADED HEAD SAW. THE CURVED TEETH HAVE HERE CUT BETWEEN THE PERFORATOR HOLES AND THE STRAIGHT TEETH BRING THE CUT NEAR THE BRAIN SURFACE. THIS IS REPEATED UNTIL THE CIRCLE IS COMPLETED AROUND THE DEPRESSED FRACTURE. DELLA CROCE'S HEAD SAW IS SHOWN HERE.

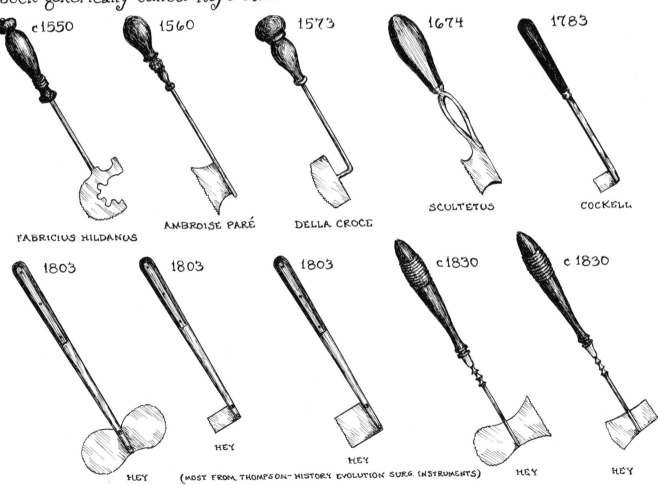

c1550 FABRICIUS HILDANUS

1560 AMBROISE PARÉ

1573 DELLA CROCE

1674 SCULTETUS

1783 COCKELL

1803 HEY

1803 HEY

1803 HEY

c1830 HEY

c1830 HEY

(MOST FROM THOMPSON- HISTORY EVOLUTION SURG. INSTRUMENTS)

BRUSHES~ for sweeping the bone sawdust from the drilled skull.

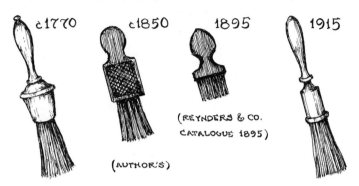

c1770   c1850   1895   1915

(REYNDERS & CO. CATALOGUE 1895)

(COMPOSITE)   (AUTHOR'S)   (KNY-SCHEERER 1915)

ELEVATORS ~ for raising the cut disc from the skull. Many included a raspatory end for filing rough bone edges.

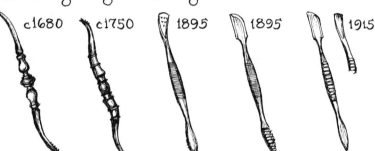

c1680   c1750   1895   1895   1915

(BENNION-ANT. MED. INSTRUMENTS)   (REYNDERS & CO. 1895)   (KNY-SCHEERER 1915)

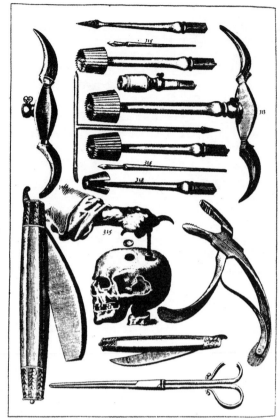

TREPHINING INSTRUMENTS FROM JOHN WOODALL'S THE SURGEONS MATE OR MILITARY & DOMESTIC SURGERY. LONDON 1639)

LENTICULARS ~ depressed the brain surface away from the trephined hole and smoothed any rough edges of the lower rim with the sharp lenticular knife edge.

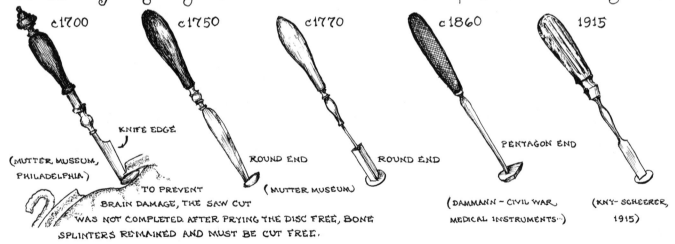

c1700   c1750   c1770   c1860   1915

KNIFE EDGE

(MUTTER MUSEUM, PHILADELPHIA)

ROUND END   ROUND END   PENTAGON END

TO PREVENT BRAIN DAMAGE, THE SAW CUT WAS NOT COMPLETED. AFTER PRYING THE DISC FREE, BONE SPLINTERS REMAINED AND MUST BE CUT FREE.

(MUTTER MUSEUM)   (DAMMANN - CIVIL WAR MEDICAL INSTRUMENTS)   (KNY-SCHEERER, 1915)

In conclusion, Gillies and Millard summed up the changing world of medical antiques in their Principles and Art of Plastic Surgery. "There is little that can be called original since a sharp flint opened an abscess and some horsehair threaded through the first thorn needle sewed up a wound. Yet all goes on, bit by bit, and the wheel of progress turns just a little in any man's lifetime."

Price Guide

Price guides are akin to a blindfolded surgeon. Instinct and experience make the best of a difficult task. Although the reader may be boggled by the wide range of values, the many variables for each class of instruments make guestimates necessary.

To be considered are general condition, intact original parts, makers marks, historical connections with such as the Revolutionary or Civil War, pieces associated with well-known physicians, age, scarcity, prototypes for later instruments, and the unusual or bizarre.

Further, a dealer may make a bargain purchase or an auctioneer may know little about medical antiques. An important piece of medical history may then be owned for considerably less than the price ranges that follow.

Prices for the microscope section are by Ben Weber, a top authority on microscopes.

MICROSCOPES
Simple compass, c. 1740-1745	200-900
Wilson, c. 1702-1750	700-900
pillar, c. 1750-1830	45-1800
tripod, c. 1900	20
pillar, adjustable arm, c. 1750-1850	450-600
dissecting, c. 1745-1906	45-1200
Compound	
Hooke, 1665	5000
Marshall, 1704	5000
Culpeper 1706-1738	4500
Cuff, c. 1750	4000
Adams, c. 1746-1760	4500-5500
Martin, 1776	2800
Dollond, 1790-1820	2500
Cary, 1820	450
Jones, c. 1824	750
Lister, 1839	1900
Ross, 1843	1200
Powell & Lealand, 1843	4500
Continental style, 1885-1900	225-550
Martin drum, 1738	1200
Oberhauser, 1840	250
Leitz, c. 1885	125
Zeiss, 1891	150
American Design	
Holmes, 1873	850
Spencer, c. 1840-1850	750-2500
Grunow, 1855	950
Tolles, 1867	450
Bulloch, 1884	400
Baush & Lomb, c. 1893-1930	125-250
Spencer, c. 1904	100
Riddells, 1853	1200
Smith, 1855	900

PLEXIMETERS
(rare)	50-100

PERCUSSORS/REFLEX HAMMERS
Whalebone, English, 1850's	70-90
1860 varieties	75-90
1900-1920	8-20

STETHOSCOPES
Monaural, wood	150-220
ivory removable ear piece	240-260
flexible	100-175
metal, 1900	100-140
binaural	
Cammann style, 1852	200-250
Palmer, Denison, 1885	140-250
Gowan, 1885	120-150
Ford, 1885	25-60
O'Kelly, Shepard, Sanson, 1895-1900	25-60
Oertel, 1915	50-85
bell chest piece, early 1900's	20-35
Phonendoscope, 1894	120-200
diaphragms, 1900	15-35
Bowles-Pilling, 1912	25-40
Jefferson, 1912	25-30
Sprague-Bowles, 1926	15-25
Meredith, 1928	15-25

BLOOD PRESSURE INSTRUMENTS
Marey wrist sphygmograph, 1857	900-1500
Dudgeon sphygmograph, 1890	400-600
Leonard Hill sphygmometer, 1885	100-125
Riva-Rocci sphygmomanometer, 1895	500-800
Janeway, 1902	200-300
Cook, 1903	200-300
Oliver, manometer, 1910	150-250
Mercer, 1911	125-220
Nicholson, 1912	125-215
Stanton, 1912	125-220
Faught, 1909-1912	125-220
Baumometer, 1917	125-200
wall, 1919	75-150
desk, 1921	75-160
Becton Dickson, 1926	75-160
pocket, 1926	75-140
Von Basch, 1887	300-450
Potain, 1889	300-400
Von Reklinghausen, 1908	250-350
Pachon, 1909	500-650
Faught, 1912	100-175
Dr. Rogers, 1900's	25-60
Tycos office, 1925	45-60
desk, 1937	40-55
hand, 1956	35-40
wall, 1961	30-40
aneroid, 1963	18-25

ELECTRO CARDIOGRAPHS	
Hindle, 1921	550-700
Cambridge, 1928-9	200-300
Beck-Lee, 1930	150-200
Victor, 1930	150-200
Beck-Lee, post war	100-150
1960 portables	60-120
OPHTHALMOSCOPES	
Helmholtz, 1850	400-550
Epkins, 1851	125-150
Ruefe, 1852	400-500
Helmholtz with Rekoss disc, 1852	200-300
Coccius, 1854	200-300
Stellwag von Carion, 1854	200-300
Liebreich, 1855	200-300
Loring, 1870's	175-250
Morton chain of lenses style, 1883	100-200
May, 1900	45-85
electric, 1900-1920	45-85
1920-1940	35-75
TONOMETERS	
Rubino, 1910	40-50
Schiotz style, 1920's	40-50
Bailliart, 1920's	50-60
OTOSCOPES	
specula, simple, set of 3, 1860-1930	15-30
bivalve, 1860-1900	18-30
1900-1915	15-25
reflector (Brunston type), 1880's	100-175
electric	
Brunton, 1895	90-175
Park, 1889	90-180
1915-1920	35-75
pneumatic	
1850's	150-200
1864-1925	25-45
HEAD MIRRORS	
1900-1920	30-45
electric lamp, 1900-1915	35-60
NASAL SPECULA	
Simple and bivalve	
1800-1860	20-30
1870-1920's	8-22
TONGUE DEPRESSORS	
1700-early 1800's, silver	100-150
horn/ivory early 1800's	20-35
metal, 1840-1890	15-35
1900 on	8-18
LARYNGOSCOPE	
Kirstein, 1895	40-60
Yankauer, 1910	50-80
Tucker, 1910	50-80
Jackson, 1924	30-40
BRONCHOSCOPES	
Killian, 1898	50-70
Jackson, 1902	50-60
1920	35-50
GASTROSCOPES	
Lerche, 1915	35-50
Kausch, 1929	35-50
VAGINAL SPECULA	
bivalves, 1700's	500-750

cylindrical, 1816-1860	150-300
valvular, 1818-1837	150-450
Cusco, 1850	30-60
Sims, 1845	65-85
later	10-25
Notts, 1870	200-300
Graves, 1878	75-125
1900-1915	30-150
RECTAL INSTRUMENTS	
1600's-1700's	300-400
Weiss	150-185
1850-1890	100-200
Desormeux, 1870	350-400
Brunton, 1880	350-400
Hilton, 1875	25-35
Brinkerhoff, 1880	25-35
1880-1927	8-50
SIGMOIDOSCOPE	
Bodenhamer, 1889	150-210
Kelly, 1908	10-40
Lynch, 1915	25-75
Tuttle, 1915	45-60
Martin-Hirschman, 1925	18-35
Montague, 1946	15-30
CATHETERS	
Solingen spiral, 1700's	90-110
silver, 1800-1840	15-25
plated 1840 on	5-15
CYSTOSCOPE	
Bozzini, 1805	2000-3000
Desormeaux, 1853	900-1400
Fisher, 1827	800-1200
Nitze, 1876	200-300
later models	75-125
Newman, 1883	150-225
Otis-Brown, 1900	75-135
SPIROMETER	
Hutchinson, 1846	700-900
Brown, 1889	250-450
Barnes, 1895	250-350
Boulitte, 1915	100-150
Simplex, 1915	40-90
THERMOMETERS	
1800	170-225
1860's	150-200
1870-80's	80-150
Immisch surface	150-225
MEDICINE CHESTS	
1700's	1000-1600
1800-60's	400-1000
field, 1800	250-275
1900	180-200
homeopathic	85-150
SURGICAL CASES	
Revolutionary capital	3000-5000
Civil War, minor	1000-1500
capital	1500-2600
pocket cases, 1860-1900	65-500
trephining set, Civil War	1500
SURGICAL WALLETS	
1825	500-600
medical/surgical, Civil War	85-400

POUCH

obstetrical, 1855 — 300-500

POCKET MEDICAL

1870-1890 — 40-50
1890-1930 — 20-35

BAGS

saddle, 1800-1860 — 300-450
homeopathic, 1840 — 190-220
1880 — 90-110
medical/surgical M.D., 1860 — 70-100
1880-1920 — 25-65

FORCEPS-DRESSING, TISSUE, SPLINTER

1700's — 90-300
1800-1860 — 35-55
1870-1900 — 15-25

FORCEPS, ARTERY

1800-1860 — 20-45
1870-1920 — 6-15

NEEDLE HOLDERS

1800 — 75-90
1880-1900 — 20-50
1900 on — 8-20

BULLET EXTRACTORS

crane/duck bill, 1500's — 200-500
1600's — 700-1000
1700's — 500-600
1800's — 60-250

OBSTETRICAL

perforators
1750 — 200-300
1800's — 70-200
crochets, 1800's — 90-170
blunt hooks, 1880's — 75-125
levers, 1800's — 90-120
cephalotribes, 1800's — 200-250
cranioclasts, 1860's — 200-250
forceps
1700's — 500-1000
1800-60 — 150-400
1870-80 — 100-250
1880-1920 — 15-50

SCISSORS

1600's — 250-300
1700's — 200-250
1800-1865 — 35-50
1870-1900 — 5-15

SCALPELS, BISTOURIES, ABSCESS, TENOTOMES

1600's — 300-350
1700's — 50-75
1800's
tortoise, folding — 22-45
ivory handle — 18-45
ebony — 12-30

lancets, spear point, 1880's — 18-45
1900's — 4-15

BLEEDING BOWLS

pewter, incised handle, 1800 — 650-850
glazed pottery, 1850 — 120-200

BLEEDING INSTRUMENTS

fleams, horn handle, c. 1860's — 40-60
brass handle — 35-60
thumb lancets, 1800's — 22-45
spring lancets, late 1700's-1800's — 90-140
cups
glass, 1700-early 1800's, pontil — 15-40
glass mid-1800's, no pontil — 8-20
teapot lamp — 40-60
sets with scarificators — 600-1100
Bauncheidt's Lebenswecker — 300-400
scarificators
octagonal brass, 1800's — 180-220
nickle plated cylindrical, c. 1870's — 125-180
syringe-cup combination set, 1800-1900 — 700-900
artificial leech, Heurteloup, set — 900-1000
leech jars
cylindrical, earthenware, c. 1860 — 800-1150
glass, short stem, c. 1840 — 300-450
urn, tall neck, perforated lid, 1800's — 2300-4000
single leech carrier, silver, 1800's — 350-400
glass, bowl-shaped, extended lip, 1800's
various sizes, pontil — 60-350
leech tubes — 35-50

VACCINATORS

tortoise shell, folding with prongs, 1870's — 55-65
with point, 1860-70 — 55-65
metal, pencil shape, lancet end — 24-28
ivory handle and blade, c. 1820 — 55-70

TOURNIQUETS

Petit, 1718-1900 — 60-150

AMPUTATION INSTRUMENTS

knives
1700's — 100-250
chany handles, 1800's — 32-70
1880-1915 all metal — 15-25
saws
bow, blacksmith-wrought, c. 1800 — 120-150
1700's, fancy frame — 900-1200
1800's, bow or tenon — 100-240
1890-1915 all metal — 25-50
chain, c. 1840 — 120-160

TREPANS

1700's — 2000-2500

TREPHINES

1700's — 400-500
1800's — 150-240
1880-1900 — 60-100

American Medical, Dental and Apothecary Museums

ALABAMA

Dr. Francis Medical and Apothecary Museum, 100 Gayle St., Jacksonville, AL 36265. The 1850 office and apothecary of Dr. Francis displays medical equipment and furniture of the period. Shown by appointment, 205-435-7203. No charge.

Landmarks Foundation, 310 N. Hull St., Montgomery, AL 36104. 12 historic houses including 1892 doctor's office, Mon.-Sat. 9:30-4, Sundays and holidays 1:30-3:30. Closed New Years, Thanksgiving, Christmas. Charge.

Thomas E. McMillan Museum, Jefferson Davis College, Alco Drive, Brewton, AL 36426. General exhibits plus mid-19th century medical, dental and pharmaceutical instruments. Mon.-Fri. 9-5. Closed New Years, Memorial Day, Labor Day, Thanksgiving, Christmas. No charge.

ARIZONA

Phoenix Baptist Hospital Museum with extensive medical artifacts in lobby. Open 24 hours daily.

Sharlot Hall Museum, 415 West Gurley St., Prescott, AZ 86301. General and medical. May-October, Tues.-Sat. 9-5, Sun. 1-5, Nov.-April, Tues.-Sat. 10-4, Sun.1-5. Closed New Years, Thanksgiving, Christmas. No charge.

Tombstone Courthouse State Historical Park, 219 Toughnut St., Tombstone, AZ 85638. General, including medical. Daily 8-5, closed Christmas. Charge.

ARKANSAS

The Castle and Museum at Inspiration Point, Highway 62, 5½ miles west, Eureka Springs, AR 72632. General, including early medical and dental equipment. Mid-April-Oct. Daily 9-5. Charge.

Jacksonport Courthouse Museum, Jacksonport State Park, Jacksonport, AR 72075. General, including medical instruments. Tues.-Sat. 8-5, Sun. 1-5, winter Tues.-Sun. 1-5. Charge.

Old Fort Museum, 320 Rogers Ave., Fort Smith, AR 72901. General, with 1920 drug store. Sept.-May, Tues.-Sat., 10-5, Sun. 1-5, June-Aug. daily 9-5. Closed New Years, Thanksgiving, Christmas. Charge.

Robinson Farm Museum & Heritage Center, Rt. 1 Box 324, Everton, AR 72633. Ozarkia materials from 19th century, including medical and dental. Closed major holidays. Charge.

Shiloh Museum, 118 W. Johnson Ave., Springdale, AR 72764. General, including medical instruments. Nov.-May, Mon.-Sat. 10-5, June-Oct., Mon.-Sat. 10-5, Sun. 1-5. Closed New Years, Thanksgiving, Christmas. No charge.

CALIFORNIA

Fullerton Arboretum, Yorba Linda Blvd. & Associated Road, Fullerton, CA 92634. Home and office of Dr. George Clark moved to site with equipment, office and pharmacy. Also general collections. Daily 8-4:45, Sun. 2-4. Closed New Years, Easter, Christmas. No charge.

Library of Los Angeles County Medical Association, 634 S. Westlake Ave., Los Angeles, CA 90057. Extensive medical museum of old medical and surgical instruments, rare medical books, pre-Columbian pottery figures, medical charicatures and prints. Mon.-Fri. 8:30-5. Closed national holidays. No charge.

Museum of Dentistry, 295 S. Flower St., Orange, CA 92668. Dental museum with equipment and artifacts dating from 1700. By appointment. Closed holidays. No charge.

Rialto Historical Society, 201-205 N. Riverside Ave., Rialto, CA 92376. General collections including medical equipment. Thurs.-Sat. 2-4. No charge.

Sacramento Valley Museum Association, Inc., 1491 E. St., Williams, CA 95987. Historic houses including apothecary shop. Mon.-Wed., Fri.-Sun. 10-5. Closed Christmas. Charge.

COLORADO

Gilpin County Historical Society Museum, P.O. Box 244, Central City, CO 80427. Historic houses with drug store replica. Daily 11-5. Closed Labor Day to Memorial Day. Charge.

CONNECTICUT

Friends Museum of the University of Connecticut Health Center, 35 S. High St., New Britain, CT 06051. Dental antiques museum. Mon.-Fri. 9-4, Sat. 9-12. Closed Legal holidays. No charge.

The Historical Museum of Medicine and Dentistry, 230 Scarborough St., Hartford, CT 06105. Extensive medical and dental displays, including the Horace Wells rooms and the discovery of anesthesia in 1844, dental office and medical instruments. Telephone 203-236-5613.

New Canaan Historical Society, 13 Oenoke Ridge, New Canaan, CT 06840. 1845 Cody Drug store is one of the historical buildings. Wed.-Thurs., Sun. 2-4. Charge.

Noank Historical Society, Inc. 17 Sylvan St., Noank, CT 06340. General and some medical. July-Aug., Wed., Sat., Sun. 2-5. No charge.

Yale Medical Library, 333 Cedar St., New Haven, CT 06510. Library, graphics, weights and measures, medical instruments, historical pharmacy. Mon.-Fri. 8:30 a.m.-12 midnight, Sat. 8:30 a.m.-10 p.m.,

Sun. and holidays 11:00 a.m.-midnight. Closed Christmas. No charge.

DISTRICT OF COLUMBIA

Armed Forces Medical Museum of the Armed Forces Institute of Pathology, Building 54, Rm. G061, Washington, D.C. 20306. Gross pathology collection, famous Billings microscope collection, and medical antiques. Mon.-Fri. 10-5, Sat.-Sun. 12-5. Closed New Years, Thanksgiving, Christmas. No charge.

National Museum of American History, 14th St. and Constitution Ave., NW, Washington, DC 20560. Extensive medical collection and displays. Daily 10-5:30. Closed Christmas. No charge.

FLORIDA

Pioneer Park Museum, Highway and State Road 64, Zolfo Springs, FL 33890. General, including medical. Sat.-Sun. 1-5:30. No charge.

Science Center of Pinellas County, 7701 22nd Ave. N, St. Petersburg, FL 33710. Varied science collections, including medicine. Oct.-May, Mon.-Sat. 9-4, June-Sept. Mon.-Fri. 9-4. Closed last 2 weeks of August, Thanksgiving and Christmas. No charge.

GEORGIA

Carter-Coile Country Doctors Museum, Bolton Drive, Winterville, GA 30683. Medical museum in 1874 office of Drs. Carter and Coile with medical equipment, anatomical exhibits. Call for appointment 404-742-5891. No charge.

Crawford W. Long Medical Museum, U.S. Highway 129, Jefferson, GA 30549. On site of the first operation using ether, performed by Dr. Crawford W. Long, and collections concerning the discovery of anesthetics. Tues.-Sat. 10-5, Sun. 2-5. Closed New Years, July 4th, Labor Day, Memorial Day, Thanksgiving and Christmas. No charge.

Georgia Agrirama—The State Museum of Agriculture, Interstate 75, Exit 20 at 8th St., Tifton, GA 31793. Varied houses and collections, including 1887 doctor's office. Winter, Sat. 9-5, Sun. 12:30-5. Summer daily 9-6. Closed New Years, Thanksgiving, Dec. 22-25. Charge.

Parks, Recreation and Historic Sites, Division of Georgia Dept. of Natural Resources, 270 Washington St. SW, Atlanta, GA 30334. General collections, including medicine. Tues.-Sat. 9-5, Sun. 2-5:30. Closed Thanksgiving, Christmas. Charge.

Westville Village Museum, Troutman Road, Lumpkin, GA 31815. Historic houses, including 1845 doctor's office. Mon.-Sat. 10-5, Sun. 1-5. Closed New Years, Thanksgiving, Christmas. Charge.

IDAHO

Twin Falls County Museum, Rt 2, Filer, ID 83328. Varied collections plus doctor's equipment. Tues., Thurs.-Sun. 10-5, Wed. 10-9. Closed holidays. Donations accepted.

ILLINOIS

International Museum of Surgical Science and Hall of Fame, 1524 N. Lake Shore Dr., Chicago, IL 60610. Medical collection showing the growth and perfection of many surgical specialties such as obstetrics, gynecology, orthopedics, urology, radiology, X-ray, heart research and acupuncture. Has Hall of Fame

and manuscript collections. Tues.-Sat. 10-4, Sun. 11-5. Closed New Years, Labor Day, Thanksgiving, Christmas. No charge.

Iroquois County Historical Society Museum, Old Courthouse, 2nd and Cherry, Watseka, IL 60970. General collections include medical instruments and apothecary items. May-Sept., Mon.-Fri. 10-4:30, Sat.-Sun. 1-4, Oct.-April, Mon.-Fri. 12-4:30, Sat.-Sun. 1-4. No charge.

Naper Settlement, 201 W. Porter Ave., Naperville, IL 60540. Historic buildings, including c.1850 Dr. Daniels house. May 5-Nov.3, Sat.-Sun. 1:30-4:30. Closed Memorial Day, Labor Day. Charge.

The Pearson Museum, 801 N. Rutledge, Springfield, IL 62708. Early American 20th century artifacts relating to medical and pharmaceutical practices, medical pre-Columbian artifacts, medical literature and art. Mon-Fri. 12-1. No charge.

Vermilion County Museum Society, 116 N. Gilbert St., Danville, IL 61832. Varied collections, including 1860s doctor's office and 1920 dental office. Tues.-Sat. 10-5, Sun., holidays 1-5. Closed Thanksgiving and Christmas. Charge.

Wood Library-Museum of Anesthesiology, 515 Busse Hwy., Park Ridge, IL 60068. Medical museum with historical equipment and anesthesiology manuscripts. Mon.-Fri. 9-4:30. Closed holidays. No charge.

INDIANA

Archives and Company Museum-Eli Lilly and Company, Lilly Center, 893 S. Delaware, Indianapolis, IN 46206. The pharmacology museum is housed in a replica of the original Lilly laboratory. Displays illustrate the pharmaceutical industry and early medicine. Mon.-Fri. 8-4. Closed national holidays. No charge.

Brown County Museum, Museum Lane, Nashville, IN 47448. Buildings and collections feature a completely equipped early doctor's office. Mon.-Oct. Sat.-Sun. 1-5. Charge.

Clinton County Museum, 301 E. Clinton St., Frankfort, IN 46041. General, including medical instruments, April-Dec., Sat.-Sun. 1:30-4:30. No charge.

Grover Museum, 52 W. Broadway, Shelbyville, IN 46176. Includes medical instruments. Sat.-Sun. 1-4. Closed holidays. No charge.

Historic Madison, Inc., 500 West St. Madison, IN 47250. Collections, including Dr. Wm. Hutching's office and hospital with early 19th century furnishings. May-Oct., Mon.-Sat. 10-4:30, Sun. 1-4:30. Charge.

IOWA

Calhoun County Historical Society, 868 8th St., Rockwell City, IA 50579. General with medical and dental equipment. June-Aug., Sundays 2-4. No charge.

Chickasaw County Historical Society Museum, Bradford Village, East on Hwy. 346, Nashua, IA 50658. Historical buildings include Dr. Pitts medical office. Memorial Day-Labor Day daily 9-5. Charge.

Floyd County Historical Museum, 500 Gilbert St., Charles City, IA 50616. General with medical and pharmacology exhibits, dental office and medical rooms. June-Aug., Thurs.-Sun. 1-4:30, May-Sept., Sat.-Sun. 1-4:30. Charge.

Grout Museum of History and Science, 503 South St., Waterloo, IA 50701. General, including apothecary shop. 10-4:30, Sat. 1-4. Labor Day-May, Tues.-Fri. 1-4:30, Sat. 1-4. Closed national holidays. No charge.

Mitchell County Historical Museum, N. 6th, Osage, IA 50461. General with medical instruments. May-Sept., Sat.-Sun. 2-5. No charge.

Wapello County Historical Museum, 402 Chester Ave., Ottumwa, IA 52501. General and early 1900 doctor's office. Mid-April-Oct., Tues.-Sun. 1:30-4:30. Charge.

KANSAS

Chisholm Trail Museum, 502 N. Washington, Wellington, KS 67152. Displays, including doctor's office. June-Aug., Tues.-Sun. 2-4, Sept.-May, Sat.-Sun. 2-4. No charge.

Cloud County Historical Museum, 635 Broadway, Concordia, KS 66901. General with some medical. Daily 1-5. No charge.

Douglass Historical Museum, 312-314 S. Forest, Douglass, KS 67039. General with doctor's office. Mon., Wed., Fri. 9:30-1:30. Closed Christmas and New Years. No charge.

Finney County Kansas Historical Society, Inc., Finnup Park, South 4, Garden City, KS 67846. General with early dental office equipment. Mid-May—mid-Sept., daily 1-5, mid-Sept.—mid-May, Sat.-Sun. 2-5. No charge.

Jewell County Historical Museum, Main St. Mankato, KS 66956. General with pharmacy and doctor's office. Thurs.-Sat. 1-4. No charge.

Kansas Health Museum. 309 Main St., Halstead, KS 67056. Medical instruments, research and movies about health. Mon.-Fri. 10-4, Sun. 1-5. Closed New Years, Easter, Memorial Day, July 4th, Labor Day, Thanksgiving and Christmas. Charge.

Kingsman County Historical Museum, 400 N. Main, Kingman, KS 67068. General exhibits, including hospital, surgical instruments and dental equipment. Fri. 9:30-4:30. Closed Christmas. No charge.

Lanesfield School Historical Society, 18745 S. Dillie Rd., Edgerton, KS 66021. General with replica of Dr. A.S. Reece's early medical office. April-Dec., Sat.-Sun., Wed. 1-5. Closed national holidays. No charge.

Meade County Historical Society Museum, 200 E. Carthage, Meade, KS 67864. Period rooms and doctor's office. Mid-May—Labor Day, Tues.-Sat. 10-12 and 1:30-5, Sun. 2-5. Labor Day—mid-May, Sat.-Sun. 2-5. Closed Thanksgiving and Christmas. No charge.

Menninger Museum and Archives, 6th St., Topeka, KS 66603. Collection of psychiatric devices such as straight jackets and cages, as well as many of Freud's manuscripts and 7 of Benjamin Rush's letters. Weekdays 9-4:30.

Old Cowtown Museum, 1871 Sim Park Dr., Wichita, KS 67203. General with two apothecary collections. March-Dec., daily 10-5, Jan.-mid-Feb., Mon.-Fri. 10-5. Charge.

Old Depot Museum, Box 145, Ottawa, KS 66067. General and dentist's office. Memorial Day-Labor Day, Sun. and holidays 1-5. No charge.

Pioneer Museum, 430 W. 4th, Ashland, KS 67831. Includes pioneer doctors and hospital equipment. May-Oct., daily 1-5, Nov.-April, daily 1-4. Closed New Years, Thanksgiving, Christmas. ? Charge.

University of Kansas Medical Center, Clendening History of Medicine Library, Rainbow at 39th St., Kansas City, KS 66103. Microscopes, Egyptian amulets, surgical instruments such as amputation sets, bleeding bowls, and instruments, obstetrical forceps, diagnostic dolls, etc. Mon.-Fri. 8-4:30. Closed New Years, Easter, July 4th, Labor Day, Thanksgiving, Christmas. ?Charge.

Wabaunsee County Historical Museum, Missouri and Third Sts., Alma, KS 66401. Displays include old doctor's office. Tues.-Sat. 10-12 and 1-4, Sun. and holidays 1-4. Closed New Years, Easter, Memorial Day, Thanksgiving, Christmas. No charge.

KENTUCKY

McDowell House and Apothecary Shop, 125 S. 2nd St. Danville, KY 40422. Medical and apothecary collections housed in 1800 McDowell House and 1795 apothecary shop. Nov.-April, Tues.-Sat. 10-12 and 1-4, Sun. 2-4, March-Oct., Mon.-Sat. 10-12 and 1-4, Sun. 2-4. Closed New Years, Thanksgiving, Easter, Christmas. Charge.

Transylvania Museum, 300 N. Broadway, Lexington, KY 40508. Collections include early 19th century scientific apparatus and instruments used in teaching 19th century medicine. Mon.-Fri. 9-4. Closed national holidays. No charge.

LOUISIANA

Bayou Folk Museum, Rt.1 Box 60, Cloutierville, LA 71416. General and country doctor's office with instruments, many from Civil War. June-mid-Aug., Tues.-Fri. 10-5, Sat.-Sun. 1-5, mid-Aug.-May, Sat. and Sun. 1-5. Closed mid-Dec.-Feb. No charge.

MARYLAND

Allegany County Historical Society, Inc., 218 Washington St., Cumberland, MD 21502. General and 19th century medical instruments and equipment. May-Oct., Tues.-Sun. 1:30-4. Charge.

Clara Barton National Historic Site, 5801 Oxford Road, Glen Echo, MD 20812. Museum in home of Clara Barton, founder of the American Red Cross. Memorabilia. Daily 10-5. Closed New Years, Thanksgiving, Christmas. No charge.

The Montgomery County Historical Society, Inc., 103 W. Montgomery Avenue, Rockville, MD 20850. General, including Stonestreet Medical Museum and 1850 doctor's office. Tues.-Sat. 12-4, first Sunday each month 2-5. Closed major holidays. Charge.

Museum of the Baltimore College of Dental Surgery, Dental School, University of Maryland at Baltimore. Early dental instruments and equipment. Mon.-Thurs. 8:30 a.m.-8:45 p.m., Fri. 8:30-5. Closed school holidays. No charge.

William P. Didusch Museum of the American Urological Association. Temporarily closed, the American

Urological Association, 1120 N. Charles St., Baltimore, MD 21201 may be contacted for future opening date. Extensive urological collections and original art work by William P. Didusch.

MASSACHUSETTS
Museum of Science, Science Park, Boston, MA 02114. Collections include history of use of ether, anatomy, body chemistry, blood, DNA, etc. Sept.-April, Tues.-Thurs. 9-4, Fri. 9-10, Sat. 9-5, Sun. 10-5. May-July, Mon.-Thurs. 9-4, Fri. 9-10, Sat. 9-5, Sun. 10-5. Closed Thanksgiving, Christmas. Charge.

Northborough Historical Society, Inc., 52 Main St., Northborough, MA 01532. General, including apothecary supplies. Mid-May-Sept., Wed. 2-4. No charge.

Old Sturbridge Village, Sturbridge, MA 01566. Outdoor living history museum with over 40 buildings. Scientific and medical equipment displays. April-Oct., daily 9-5, Nov.-March, Tues.-Sun. 10-4. Closed New Years, Christmas. Charge.

MICHIGAN
Allegan County Historic Museum, 113 Walnut, Allegan, MI 49010. General, including dental and medical equipment. June-Aug., Fri. 2-5. No charge.

Bernard Historical Society Museum, 1 North Harbor St., Grand Haven, MI 49417. General with medical instruments and includes 1933 brick hospital. June-Sept., Sun. 1-5, July-Aug., daily 1-5. No charge.

Mackinac Island State Park Commission, Box 370, Mackinac, Island, MI 49757. Historic buildings, including Dr. William Beaumont building, reconstructed 1954 and his experiments on gastric physiology. Daily 9-6 on Mackinac Island. May-mid-June and Labor Day-mid-Oct. Charge.

Mecosta County Historical Museum, Elm and Stewart, Big Rapids, MI 49307. General with pharmacy display. April-Oct., Fri. 2-6. No charge.

Monroe County Historical Museum, 126 S. Monroe St., Monroe, MI 48161. Custer artifacts, also medical and dental equipment. May-Sept., Tues.-Sun. 10-5, Oct.-April, Thurs.-Sun. 10-5. Closed Easter, Thanksgiving, Christmas. No charge.

Montague Museum and Historical Association, Church and Meade Sts., Montague, MI 49437. General and doctor's office. Sat.-Sun. 1-5. No charge.

Museum of Arts and History, 1115 Sixth St., Port Huron, MI 48060. General and surgeon's instruments from Ft. Gratiot, 1814-1879. Wed.-Sun. 1-4:30. Closed national holidays. No charge.

Sanilac Historical Museum, 228 S. Ridge St., Port Sanilac, MI 48469. General collections with some medical. Mid-June-Labor Day, Thurs.-Sun. 1-4:30, Labor Day-Sept., Sat. and Sun. 1-4:30. Charge.

Tri-Cities Historical Society Museum, 1 North Harbor St., Grand Haven, MI 49417. General and medical. May-Sept., Wed.-Sun. 2-10. Charge.

MINNESOTA
Bakken Museum of Electricity in Life, 3537 Zenith Avenue S., Minneapolis, MN 55416. Tel: 612-927-6508. Extensive displays of electrotherapy in medicine. Write for details.

Dakota County Historical Society, 130 3rd Avenue N., S. St. Paul, MN 55075. Collections include drug store and dental office. Tues.-Fri. 8-4:30, Sat. 8-1. Closed national holidays. No charge.

Mayo Medical Museum, Mayo Foundation, 200 First St. SW, Rochester, MN 55905. Exhibits and models illustrating biology of man, medical and surgical problems, care and treatment. Mon.-Fri. 9-9. Sat. 9-5, Sun. 1-5. Closed New Years, Easter, Memorial Day, July 4th, Labor Day, Thanksgiving, Christmas. No charge.

Wright County Historical Society, 101 Lake Blvd., Buffalo, MN 55313. General and early medical apparatus. Mon.-Fri. 8-4:30. No charge.

MISSISSIPPI
Amory Regional Museum, 3rd St. & 8th Ave.S., Amory, MS 38821. General with medical instruments and equipment of Dr. B.C. Tubb—who practiced longer than any other physician in Monroe County. Mon.-Fri. 9-5, Sat.-Sun. 1-5. Closed New Years, Memorial Day, July 4th, Labor Day, Thanksgiving, Christmas. No charge.

The Florence McLeod Hazard Museum, 316 7th St.N., Columbus, MS 39701. General with medical instruments. Mon.-Fri. 9-5, Sat.-Sun. 1-5. Closed New Years, Memorial Day, July 4th, Labor Day, Thanksgiving, Christmas. No charge.

Marshall County Historical Museum, 220 E. College Ave., Holly Springs, MS 38635. General and physician's office exam room equipment.

University Museums, The University of Mississippi, University, MS 38677. General including surgical instruments. Tues.-Sat. 10-4, Sun. 1-4. No charge.

MISSOURI
Clay County Historical Museum, 14 N. Main, Liberty, MO 64068. General displays and medical and druggist equipment housed in an 1877 drug store. Tues.-Sat. 1-4, Sun. 1-4. Closed national holidays. No charge.

Friends of Arrow Rocks, Inc., Arrow Rocks, MO 65320. Historic houses and Dr. John Sappington Museum and 1840 Pioneer Doctor's Museum. Memorial Day-Labor Day, Mon. and Sat. 10, 1:30 and 3, Sun. 1:30 and 3 tours.

National Museum of Medical Quackery of the St. Louis Medical Historical Museum, 3839 Lindell Blvd., St. Louis, MO 63108. Full range of quackery and frauds. Weekdays from 11-4. ?No charge.

Pattee House Museum, 1202 Penn St., St. Joseph, MO 64502. General with apothecary and dental office exhibits. June-Labor Day, Mon.-Sat. 10-5, Sun. and holidays 1-5. April-May and Sept.-Dec. Sat.-Sun. 1-5. Christmas Day 1-5. No charge.

St. Louis Science Center, 5050 Oakland Avenue, St. Louis, MO 63110. General science including medical collections. June-Aug., Mon. Tues. 9:30-5, Wed.-Sat. 9:30-9, Sun. 12-5. Sept.-May, Mon.-Thurs. 9:30-5, Fri. Sat. 9:30-8, Sun. 12-5. Closed New Years, Thanksgiving, Christmas. No charge.

MONTANA
Blaine County Museum, 501 Indiana, Chinook, MT 59523. Local exhibits and dentist's office. May-Sept. 30, Tues.-Sat. 8-5, Sun. 2-4:30. No charge.

Copper Village Museum, 110 E. 8th St., Aneconda, MT 59711. Local history and bottle collection from first drug store in town, antique doctor's furniture and books, diplomas of Dr. W.E. Long. Tues.-Thurs. 10-12, 1-3, Sat. Sun. 1-4. Closed legal holidays. No charge.

Liberty County Museum, Chester, MT 59522. Local, military and medical displays. Memorial Day-Labor Day, daily 2-5 and 7-9. No charge.

Mondak Heritage Center, 120 Third Ave. SE, Sidney, MT 59270. Village includes dentist's office. Call for hours 406-482-3500. No charge.

NEBRASKA

Brownville Historical Society Museum, Main St., Brownville, NE 68321. General with dental office. June-Aug., daily 1-5, May-Oct., Sun. 1-5. Charge.

Gage County Historical Museum, 2nd and Court, Highway 4 and 136 West, Beatrice, NE 68310. Local collections including 1900's X-ray machine, medical, dental equipment, June-Aug., Tues.-Fri. 1-5, Sun. 1:30-5. Sept.-May, Tues.-Thurs. 1-5, Sun. 1:30-5. Closed Easter, Thanksgiving, Christmas. No charge.

Heritage House Museum, 107 Clinton, Weeping Water, NE 68463. Includes 1800's medical books, medical instruments and drugs, original 1880 office at Dr. Jesse Fate. April-Oct., Sun. 2-5. No charge.

Otoe County Museum, 230 Elm, Syracuse, NE 68446. Displays include doctor's office. April-Dec., Sun. 2-5. No charge.

NEW HAMPSHIRE

Durham Historic Association Museum, Newmarket Road and Main St., Durham, NH 03824. Local history and doctor's equipment. June-Aug., Tues.-Sat. 1-4. No charge.

NEW YORK

The Arnold and Marie Schwartz College of Pharmacy and Health Sciences, 75 De Kalb Avenue, Brooklyn, NY 11201. Pharmacy artifacts, documents, drugs, glassware, jars and related pharmacy materials. Winter Mon.-Fri. 9-5. Summer, Mon.-Thurs. 9-5:30. Closed national holidays. No charge.

Cayuga Museum of History and Art, 203 Genesee St., Auburn, NY 13021. General with medical instruments. Tues.-Fri. 1-5, Sat. 9-12 and 1-5, Sun. 2-5. Closed New Years, Labor Day, Thanksgiving, Christmas. No charge.

Cornell Medical School, 1300 York Ave., New York, NY 10001. The faculty room contains the remarkable medical collection of Dr. Philip Reichert with emphasis on medical diagnostic instruments and apparatus. Permission is necessary. No charge.

Museum Village in Orange County, Museum Village Rd., Monroe, NY 10950. The 38 buildings include an apothecary shop. Mid-April-Oct., Tues.-Sun. 10-5. Charge.

Rochester Museum and Science Center, 657 East Avenue, Box 1480, Rochester, NY 14603. Collections include those of the "medical industry". Mon.-Sat. 9-5, Sun. and holidays 1-5. Closed Christmas. Charge.

Thousand Island Old Town Hall Museum, 401 Riverside Dr., Old Town Hall, Clayton, NY 13624. Village square of historical houses including a drug store. June-Sept., daily 10-5. No charge.

NORTH CAROLINA

Beaufort Historical Association, Box 1709, Beaufort, NC 28516. Historical houses include 1796 apothecary shop. Mon.-Sat. 9:30-4:30, Summer, Sun. 2-4. Closed Easter, Thanksgiving, Christmas. Charge.

The Country Doctor Museum, Vance St., Bailey, NC 27807. 18th, 19th and early 20th century medicine and pharmaceuticals are housed in the 1857 Dr. Freeman office and the 1887 Dr. Brantley office. Sun.-Wed. 2-5. No charge.

Davidson County Historical Museum, Old Court House on the Square, Lexington, NC 27292. General including dental equipment. Tues.-Fri. 10-4, Sun. 2-4. Closed holidays. No charge.

Greensboro Historical Museum, Inc., 130 Summit Ave., Greensboro, NC 27401. Late 19th century village exhibit includes drug store and doctor's office. Tues.-Sat. 10-5, Sun. 2-5. Closed New Years, Easter, Thanksgiving, Christmas. No charge.

North Carolina Division of History, 109 E. Jones St., Raleigh, NC 27611. General including medicine. Tues.-Sat. 8-5:30, Sun. 1-6. Closed national holidays. No charge.

Trent Collection in the History of Medicine, Duke University Medical Center Library, Durham, NC 27710. Large collection of medical and scientific books. No museum. Mon.-Fri. 8:30-5. No charge.

NORTH DAKOTA

Fort Seward Historical Society, Inc., 503 15th St. SE #3, Jamestown, ND 58401. General collections including medical. June-Sept., Wed., Sun. 2-5 and 7-9. No charge.

Frontier Museum, Williston, ND 58801. Historic buildings include old time doctor's and dentist's office. May-Labor Day, Sun. 1-5. Charge.

Hettinger County Historical Society, Box 176, Regent, ND 58650. 1911-1965 Dr. S.W. Hill drug store with equipment. Wed. 1-3. No charge.

OHIO

Center of Science and Industry of the Franklin County Historical Society, 280 E. Broad St., Columbus, OH 43215. General and also medical. Mon.-Sat. 10-5, Sun. 1-5:30. Closed holidays. Charge.

Dr. John Harris Dental Museum, Bainbridge, OH 45612. Dental museum housed in former office of Dr. John Harris. Mid-April-Nov.1, Fri.-Wed. 10-5. No charge.

Historic Southwest Ohio, Inc., 812 Dayton St., Cincinnati, OH 45214. Historic structures including doctor's office. Tues.-Thurs. 10-4, Sat.-Sun. 1-5. Charge.

Holmes County Historical Society, 233 N. Washington St., Millersburg, OH 44654. Has early medical furnishings. June-Nov., Thurs.-Sun. 1:30-4:30. Charge.

Howard Dittrick Museum of Historical Medicine, 11000 Euclid Ave., Cleveland, OH 44106. Medical history museum collections relate to medical practice, dentistry, pharmacy and nursing. Exhibits emphasize medicine in the 19th and early 20th century. Includes doctors' offices and a 19th century pharmacy. Mon.-Sat.10-5. Closed national holidays. No charge.

McCook House, Public Square, Carrollton, OH 44615. Includes antique medical instruments. June-mid-Oct., Fri., Sat. 10-5, Sun. 1-5. Charge.

Mercer County Historical Museum, the Riley Home, 130 E. Market, Celina, OH 45883. Includes medical, dental and health display. Wed.-Fri. 8:30-4, Sun. 1-4. Closed holidays. No charge.

The Oliver Tucker Historic Museum, State Rt. 60, Beverly, OH 45715. Has doctor's office furniture and instruments. June-Aug., Sat., Sun. 1-5. No charge.

Richland County Museum, 51 Church St., Lexington, OH 44904. Have some medical instruments. May-Oct., Sat., Sun. 1-4. No charge.

Salem Historical Society, 208 S. Broadway Ave., Salem, OH 44460. Collections including examining rooms, medical instruments and medicine bottles. Fri. 6:30-8:30, Sun. 2-4. Closed major holidays. Charge.

Wood County Historical Museum, 13660 County Home Rd., Bowling Green, OH 43402. Includes medical instruments. Wed.-Fri. 12-4, Sun. 1-4. Charge.

OKLAHOMA

Connors State College Museum, Connors State College, Warner, OK 74469. Collections including medical instruments and journals. Sept.-May, Mon.-Fri. 8-10. Closed major holidays. No charge.

Har-Ber Village, Rt.6, Box 470, Grove, OK 74344. General including doctor's office and drug store. May-Oct., daily 9-6. No charge.

OREGON

Junction City Historical Society, 655 Holly St., Junction City, OR 97448. Furnishings, medical tools, dental tools, housed in 1872-1878 house of first city doctor, Dr. Norman Lee. Fourth Sun. of the month 2-5, daily 1-8 during Scandinavian festival. No charge.

PENNSYLVANIA

Baldwin-Reynolds House Museum, 639 Terrace St., Meadville, PA 16335. General including medical instruments and historic Dr. J.R. Mosier medical office. Memorial Day-Labor Day, Wed., Sat., Sun. 1-5. Charge.

Cyclorama of Life, Lankenau Hospital, City Line and Lancaster Aves., Philadelphia, PA 19151. Human growth in development, medical history. Mon.-Fri. 9-5.?Charge.

Historical Dental Museum, Temple University School of Dentistry, 3223 N. Broadway St., Philadelphia, PA 19140. Dental museum with 1750-1930 dental equipment, furniture, instruments, paintings, documents. Mon.-Fri. 9-5. Closed New Years, Good Friday, Easter, Memorial Day, first 2 weeks of July, Labor Day, Thanksgiving, Friday after Thanksgiving, Dec. 24, 25. No charge.

Joseph Priestly House, 472 Priestly Ave., Northumberland, PA 17857. In 1794 Joseph Priestly house are antique scientific equipment and a library on Priestly. Tues.-Sat. 9-5, Sun. 12-5. Closed New Years, Martin Luther King Day, Columbus Day, Veterans' Day, Election Day, Thanksgiving, Christmas. Charge.

Mutter Museum, College of Physicians of Philadelphia, 19 S. 22nd St., Philadelphia, PA 19103. Medical museum of human anatomy and pathology, medical history, development of medical instrumentation, development of fetus and anomalies, folklore, quackery, military medicine, nursing and apothecary artifacts, memorabilia of physicians, medical antiques, medical art. Tues.-Fri. 10-4. Closed holidays. No charge.

SOUTH CAROLINA

Macaulay Museum of Dental History, Medical University of South Carolina, 171 Ashley Ave., Charleston, SC 29425. Dental museum with 6,000 items consisting of antique dental chairs, foot-powered drills, cabinets, lathe, old dental X-ray units, itinerant dentists' medicine cases, cases of molds for crowns, tooth keys and many other dental antiques. Mon.-Fri. 9-5. Closed holidays. No charge.

The Museum, 106 Main St., Greenwood, SC 29646. General including replica of doctor's office. Tues.-Fri. 9-5, Sat., Sun. 2-5. Closed legal holidays. No charge.

Walnut Grove Plantation, Rt.1 Box 200, Roebuck, SC 29376. Collections including doctor's office. Tues.-Sat. 11-5, Sun. 2-5. Closed holidays. Charge.

Waring Historical Library, Medical University of South Carolina, 171 Ashley Ave., Charleston, SC 29425. Medical objects include doctor's saddle bags, medical chests, amputation kits, electro-therapeutic machines, bleeding instruments, obstetrical specula and forceps, pharmaceutical items, manuscripts. Mon.-Fri. 9-5. Closed holidays. No charge.

SOUTH DAKOTA

Moody County Museum, East Pipestone Ave., Flandreau, SD 57028. Including early dental office. Memorial Day-Labor Day, Sun. and holidays, 2-5. No charge.

Prairie Village, P.O. Box 256, Madison, SD 57042. 40 restored buildings including dentist's office. Mid-May-Labor Day, daily 9-4, Memorial Day-Labor Day, daily 9-6. Charge.

TENNESSEE

Abraham Lincoln Museum, Lincoln Memorial University, Harrogate, TN 37752. Lincoln and Civil War material included. Civil War medical equipment laboratory. May-Oct., Mon.-Sat. 9-6, Sun. 1-6, Nov.-April, Mon.-Sat. 9-4, Sat. 9-4, Sun. 1-4. Closed New Years, Easter, Thanksgiving, Christmas. Charge.

Oakland Historic House Museum, 900 N. Maney Ave., Murfreesboro, TN 37130. Civil War cotton plantation with some medical. Tues.-Sat. 10-4:30. Sun. 1-4:30. Charge.

TEXAS

Gregg County Historical Museum, Fredonia and Bank St., Longview, TX 75606. Exhibits including dentist's office. Tues.-Sat. 10-4, Sun. 1-4. Closed major holidays. Charge.

Jefferson Historical Society and Museum, 223 Austin, Jefferson, TX 75657. General and medical. Daily and holidays, 9:30-5. Charge.

Magdalene Charlton Memorial and Griffin Memorial

House, N. Pine St., Tomball, TX 77375. Including pioneer country doctor's office. Sun. 2-5. Charge.

Museum of Medical Science, 5800 Caroline St. in Hermann Park, Houston, TX 77030. Collections including digestive and reproductive heart and lung displays, transparent manikin, etc., the 5 senses, brain and nervous systems, dental exhibit. Sun.-Mon. 12-4:45, Tues.-Sat. 9-4:45. No charge.

The Old Courthouse Museum, Old Courthouse, Peter Whetstone Square, Marshall, TX 75670. Collections include doctor's room and a dental office. Tues.-Fri. 9-5, Sat. 1:30-5. Closed New Years, Memorial Day, July 4th, Labor Day, Thanksgiving, week preceding and including Dec. 25. Charge.

Wharton County Historical Museum, 231 S. Fulton, Wharton, TX 77488. Collections including medical equipment. Tues.-Fri. 9-5. Sat., Sun. 2-5. No charge.

VERMONT

Franklin County Museum, Church St., St. Albans, VT 05478. Includes doctor's office. July-Aug., Tues.-Sat. 1-4. No charge.

Missisquoi Valley Historical Society, Main St., North Troy, VT 05859. General and medical instruments. June-Aug., Sat., Sun. 1-4. No charge.

Randolph Historical Society, Inc., Village Building., Salisbury St., Randolph, VT 05060. Collections include doctor's office. July-Aug. by appointment, 802-728-5398. Charge.

VIRGINIA

Arlington Historical Museum, 1805 S. Arlington Ridge Rd., Arlington, VA 22210. General collections with medical instruments. Fri., Sat. 11-3, Sun. 2-4. Closed holidays. No charge.

Goochland County Museum and Historical Center, Goochland, VA 23063. Collections include medical instruments. May-Oct., Mon.-Fri. 10-3. Closed holidays. No charge.

Historic Crab Orchard Museum, Rt 19-Rt 460, Tazewell, VA 24651. General with medical instruments.

Hugh Mercer Apothecary Shop, 1020 Caroline St., Fredericksburg, VA 22401. Pharmaceutical and medical implements and historic papers housed in 1761 Mercer Apothecary Shop. April-Oct., daily 9-5. Nov.-Dec., March daily 9-4, Jan.-Feb. daily 10-4. Closed New Years and Christmas. Charge.

Meadow Farm Museum, Mountain and Courtney Rds., Glen Allen, VA 23063. Includes medical instruments, books, manuscripts. Tues.-Sun. 12-4. Charge.

Spotsylvania Historic Association, Inc., P.O. Box 64, Spotsylvania County, VA 22553. Includes pharmaceutical collection. Mon.-Fri. 10-3. No charge.

Stabler-Leadbeater Apothecary Shop Museum, 105-107 S. Fairfax St., Alexandria, VA 22314. Pharmaceutical equipment with 800-900 original apothecary bottles, housed in 1792 apothecary shop. Mon.-Sat. 10-4:30. Closed holidays. No charge.

WASHINGTON

Anacortes Museum, 1305 8th, Anacortes, WA 98221. General with medical and dental instruments. Thurs.-Mon. 1-5. Closed major holidays. Donations accepted.

Chelan County Historical Museum, 5698 Museum Drive, Cashmere, WA 98815. Historic buildings including 1890 doctor's and dentist's office. April-Oct., Mon.-Sat., holidays 10-4:30, Sun. 1-4:30. No charge.

WISCONSIN

Barron County Historical Society, 1-1½ miles west of Cameron on Museum Road, Barron, WI 54812. General with dental, medical and veterinary tools, dentist's office and doctor's office. June-Labor Day, Thurs.-Sun. 1-5. No charge.

Fort Crawford Medical Museum, Stovall Hall of Health, 717 S. Beaumont Rd, Prarie du Chien, WI 53821. Medical history complex exhibited in c.1785-1853 restored Fort Crawford Military Hospital. Doctor's office, dentist's office and pharmacy of 1890's. May-Oct., daily 10-5. Charge.

Fort Winnebago Surgeons Quarters, R.R.1 Box 10, Portage, WI 53901. History museum housed in 1819 surgeons' quarters with military and medical instruments. May-Oct., daily 10-4. Charge.

Pioneer Museum, Main St., Wild Rose, WI 54984. Includes medical display and drugstore—country store.

Teeples' Thunderbird Museum, P.O. Merrillan, Hatfield, WI 54754. General with medical antiques. May-Labor Day, Tues.-Sun. and holidays 10-4. No charge.

Index